REVIEWING BASIC EMT SKILLS: A Guide for Self-Evaluation

Editorial Board

REVIEWING BASIC EMT SKILLS: A Guide for Self-Evaluation

Bertram M. Siegel, EMSI

General Editors

Richard L. Judd, PhD, EMSI
Executive Dean and Professor of Emergency
Medical Sciences, Central Connecticut State College
New Britain, Connecticut

Thomas J. Hauser, BA, EMT
Senior Editor, Emergency Training
Westport, Connecticut

Printed in the United States of America

ISBN 0-940432-00-

This text is dedicated to Myrna

and to the families of the thousands of volunteer EMS personnel. Without the understanding and support of their husbands, wives, and children, these volunteers could not provide their neighborhoods with quality pre-hospital care.

Contents

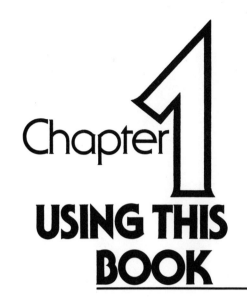

Chapter 1
USING THIS
BOOK

Using this Book

An EMT provides emergency care based on the knowledge he has obtained in his training. The body of knowledge he must retain covers a wide area, including specific facts, general concepts, and precise physical skills. All this knowledge must be learned thoroughly and permanently so it can be applied with confidence in the varied and difficult situations the EMT encounters. It must be so familiar to him that it can be recalled quickly and surely, under pressure, at a moment's notice.

Becoming this familiar with the vast amount of information an EMT must use is not an easy task. Even after thorough study, it is often difficult to determine whether or not your mastery of a subject is complete. How can you judge if you really remember all the information you might need, and if you remember it in enough detail without misunderstanding or uncertainty?

This book is designed to help you evaluate your mastery of the course material. Whether you are an EMT student or a practicing EMT, it will help you identify areas of weakness, and enable you to learn and remember the things that are not yet firmly implanted.

If you are just entering EMT work, it is impossible for you to imagine all of the many different situations that might present themselves in the field. You probably cannot even suspect the many different ways a seemingly simple situation can become complex. The questions and situations presented in this book will expose you to these hidden problems and unforeseen situations. They will present problems the way they appear to the working EMT in the field. In this way, they will allow you to evaluate your understanding of the facts, concepts, and practices that provide the basis of good emergency care.

While this book helps you identify areas of weakness in your knowledge, it will also help you overcome them by presenting the information you are lacking in a way that will help you remember it. **Reviewing Basic EMT Skills** is not a textbook. It assumes that you have thoroughly studied the content elsewhere. But mastering the content of the EMT course involves much more than simply reading textbooks and observing classroom lectures and demonstrations. To become completely comfortable with all these facts, it is necessary to use them: to answer questions with them, to relate them to other facts, and to determine the proper course of patient care. Only by constantly manipulating memorized facts will they become permanently imprinted and remain ready for rapid recall. This book will provide you with the kind of exercise that develops a lasting and useful knowledge of emergency medical procedures.

Reviewing Basic EMT Skills has been divided into chapters covering the major topics in emergency care. Within each chapter are several sections. Each will play a specific role in helping you evaluate and expand your knowledge.

Comprehensive Questions

The Comprehensive Questions at the beginning of each chapter give you an overall view of the understanding you must have by chapter's end. Each asks for a full discussion of a particular aspect of EMT work. It can only be answered if you have a thorough knowledge of the specific facts and the general principles that are at work. While the skills and facts are dealt with elsewhere, these questions ask you to explain the concepts that lie behind them. Learning these concepts is a vital part of your training. It will give you the understanding you need to apply the facts and skills intelligently in real situations. As you read these questions, understand that they are setting your goals for the unit. If you can comfortably and thoroughly answer each of them, you have a good working knowledge of the material.

It is, however, more likely that you will be uncomfortable with many of these questions. They will serve to show you where your knowledge is incomplete or unclear. That is their purpose. Rather than stopping to work on full answers to these questions, move ahead into the chapter. Consider them a framework you are trying to fill out by your further study. Then, when you have completed the chapter, return to the Comprehensive Questions and answer them again.

If when you first read the Comprehensive Questions you feel you can answer them well, don't assume the rest of the chapter will have no value for you. One of the purposes of this book is to help you locate areas where you may not realize that your knowledge is incomplete. The sections that follow will present questions and situations you may be unaware of, and will give you the ability to create a much more thorough and detailed answer to each of the Comprehensive Questions. Use the rest of the chapter, then go back to these questions and compare your new answer to your original one. The odds are great there will be a significant difference. If you remain unclear about any aspect of the material covered in the chapter, investigate it further in other sources or with your instructor or training director.

Performance Skills

The list of Performance Skills in each chapter includes the physical, manipulative tasks that are introduced. They are the things you must be able to do quickly and efficiently to provide proper patient care. Clearly a book cannot substitute for the actual practice that is necessary to master these skills and perform them well at an accident scene. Use this checklist to remind yourself of the skills you need. Go over each one in your mind, following its procedure step by step. Write out the steps if you feel it will help reinforce them. Then, at every opportunity, practice the skill itself until you can do it smoothly and with confidence.

Each individual skill is listed here only when it is first introduced, not separately under every subject area where it might be needed. Artificial ventilation, for example, is listed when it is first introduced, but not again in the chapter on CPR where it is an important component skill. In most chapters, skills learned earlier are needed along with those just being introduced.

Reference Data

The data that has been included in this section is a collection of specific facts that must be committed to memory in order to carry out the various emergency procedures. This is by no means a summary of the material covered by the chapter. General knowledge of medical principles and full understanding of emergency procedures are things which must be first learned through the use of textbooks, lectures, and demonstrations. It is assumed that these things have been studied thoroughly before use of this book is begun.

It is very possible, however, that while general principles and procedures have been learned, specific facts needed to apply them properly have been missed or forgotten. While you may be comfortable with the general procedure for artificial ventilation of an infant, the exact rate that is used may need reinforcement many times over before it is firm in your mind. What the Reference Data section provides, therefore, is a concise listing of this specific information. It serves to make you aware that these are the facts you must know and that require further study if they are not already part of your working knowledge.

Read the data carefully. Reacquaint yourself with the facts that are presented and get an idea of how thoroughly you remember them. Use this evaluation to decide what further study you need and how you should approach it.

Review Questions and Answers

These multiple-choice, short-answer questions provide the primary means of evaluating your knowledge and skills in the various areas of emergency care. They are designed to check every aspect of EMT work from general medical knowledge to the specifics of applying particular treatments. Many of these questions will present you with problems as they are encountered in actual emergency situations. You will be able to evaluate not only your ability to recall facts, but to weigh possibilities, make decisions, and draw conclusions. The questions will allow you to see very clearly how much you know, and how much you have yet to master in becoming a good EMT.

But the exercise is not just one of evaluation. It is also one of reinforcement and learning. As you read each question, think it out completely. Be certain you know exactly what is being asked and exactly what is meant by each of the possible answers. Then, when you check for the correct answer, read it thoroughly even if you know you have chosen correctly. This is one more step in firmly registering this fact in your mind. If you chose the incorrect answer, reading the explanation of the correct one will give you the information you need and help you remember it next time. Because you are actually working with the information by answering questions rather than simply reading or hearing it, it is more thoroughly absorbed and more easily recalled.

If you are at all confused by an answer, be certain to check further in your textbook or with your instructor.

Practical Applications

In this section you are given descriptions of specific situations which may present themselves to you in the field. By considering what actions you would take in these situations you can evaluate how well prepared you are to deal with real problems in emergency care.

In each situation, think about the information you are given and try to picture it clearly in your mind. Then, outline the step-by-step procedures you would follow in handling the patient. Begin with your arrival at the scene, even if it is clear that the central question being raised has to do with your action at a later stage. By always going over the early steps of patient evaluation and care, you will make them an established part of your routine.

If you come to a point in the treatment where your next step would depend on information not given in the text, such as how the patient was responding to treatment, consider what the likely possibilities are and think about how you would act in any of those cases.

This exercise is designed to help you construct situations in your mind and imagine how you would act. There are no simple, precise answers, and no answers are given. The main purpose is to evaluate whether you feel confident that you know how to handle the situation. If you feel unsure, figure out what aspect of the problem you are unsure of and clarify the proper procedure with your instructor.

Because of the content of some of the chapters, not all sub-sections appear in each one. In the chapter that describes the workings of the respiratory and circulatory systems, for example, there are no Performance Skills. This chapter is simply a source of information; it is not instructive in any particular task. There is no section of Practical Applications for the chapter on bandaging because, regardless of what situation you are in, the process of applying the bandage remains the same. For the most part, however, each of the chapter sub-sections can play an important part in helping you master the course material.

Chapter 22 deals with the use of anti-shock trousers. In many areas this skill is included in the basic level of EMT training; in others it is considered a more advanced skill. It has been included here as an optional chapter for use if this topic is part of your basic program.

Practices in emergency care are constantly scrutinized and revised. Accepted procedures are often changed, and there are often differences from one location to another regarding what is proper. If anything presented in this book appears to conflict with practice you have been taught, bring it to the attention of your instructor or training director. A full discussion of the differences will not only clarify any conflict but help you to gain a better understanding of the question involved.

Chapter 2
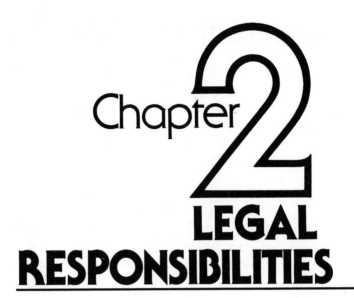

LEGAL
RESPONSIBILITIES

Comprehensive Questions

1. What are the conditions that must be met before an EMT can give emergency care? Discuss conscious patients, unconscious patients, and minors.

2. Under what conditions is the EMT prohibited from starting emergency treatment?

3. What are the obligations of an EMT who happens upon an accident scene within his local jurisdiction? outside his local jurisdiction? outside his state?

4. What responsibilities does the EMT have once he has begun treatment of a patient?

5. What are the statutes that are designed to protect the EMT from civil damages? Discuss the limitations of these statutes.

Reference Data

LEGAL CONCERNS

1. **Good Samaritan Laws** vary from state to state, but generally "hold harmless"—or protect from civil damages—those who render emergency care within the bounds of their training or license, except for gross negligence.

2. **Negligence** is a complex legal issue. Negligence must be proven. There must be evidence that the accused had a duty to act; that he failed to act as a "prudent man" would have acted under the same circumstances; that he did not act according to the standards of care expected; and that as a result of this failure, an injury occurred to the patient.

3. **The Duty to Act** doctrine requires that a public or municipal ambulance come to the aid of an injured person in that jurisdiction. Providers that do not charge for their services—including public, municipal, and volunteer services—are required to respond to every request for help.

4. **The Right to Refuse Treatment** gives any conscious, mentally competent adult the right to refuse treatment for himself, or a minor in his custody, for religious or any other reasons.

5. **Consent** must be given by a patient before the EMT may begin treatment.
   a. "Actual" or "informed" consent: The patient agrees to receive care after he is told in an understandable manner of the treatment to be performed. **With minors and mentally incompetent:** Actual consent must be given by a parent, or other adult so close to the patient as to be considered responsible, before care can be rendered.
   b. "Implied" consent: The law assumes that an unconscious patient would give his consent to receive treatment in an emergency. **With minors and mentally incompetent:** When no parent or guardian can be located to give actual consent for treatment, implied consent is assumed.

6. **Abandonment** occurs when a responder terminates the care of a patient in need of continuing care before another competent health professional has taken responsibility for the patient.

7. **Pronouncement of Death** is never made by an EMT. Only a medical examiner, or in some cases a physician, can declare death.

Review Questions

Select the correct answer for each of the following questions. There is only *one* correct answer for each.

1. An accident victim is a minor. He has a lacerated artery. What should you do if you cannot reach the parents after making an effort to do so?
   a. Telephone the physician at the emergency care center and ask for permission to proceed.
   b. Get permission from the police to proceed with treatment.
   c. Take the child to the hospital but give no treatment.
   d. Assume the parents' consent for treatment.

2. When a patient is unconscious, or so seriously injured that his judgment is impaired, you should assume that he wishes to be treated. The legal basis for this action is known as:
   a. applied consent.
   b. conditioned consent.
   c. implied consent.
   d. replied consent.

3. You arrive at the scene and the patient's husband requests that his wife be transported to the hospital. The patient is suffering severe abdominal pain, but refuses to go. Will you transport? Why?
   a. Yes; the patient needs it.
   b. No; the patient refuses.
   c. Yes; the husband requests it.
   d. No; death is not imminent.

4. The intent of Good Samaritan Laws is to:
   a. protect responders from civil damages when they stop to give emergency care as long as they act within the bounds of their training.
   b. protect a person who stops at the scene of an accident, decides he is unable to help, and leaves the scene.
   c. protect a person who stops at the scene of an accident and commits an act of gross negligence.
   d. protect victims of accidents from incompetent first aid treatment.

5. If an EMT stops to help an injured person, then leaves before other help arrives, he may be accused of:
   a. negligence.
   b. breech of duty.
   c. abandonment.
   d. malpractice.

6. You are called to an automobile accident. As an EMT you will perform all of the following functions *except one.* Which is it?
    a. Transport the patient to a hospital.
    b. Obtain all necessary information before leaving the scene.
    c. Pronounce the patient dead, if this is the case.
    d. Drive with consideration for others.

7. Which of the following professional behaviors should be performed in order to reassure an injured patient?
    a. Touch the patient gently.
    b. Explain the care you are giving to him.
    c. Inquire about current and past medical problems.
    d. All of the above.

Answers to Review Questions

1: d. You should assume the parents' consent for treatment.

2: c. Implied consent assumes that in a true emergency in which there is a significant risk of death, disability, or deterioration of condition, the unconscious or mentally incompetent patient would give his consent to treatment.

3: b. A competent patient has the right to refuse treatment. The EMT should explain why treatment and transportation to a medical facility are in the patient's best interest, but cannot force him to go to a hospital.

4: a. Good Samaritan Laws are designed to protect from civil damages those who render aid within the bounds of their training. However, they cannot and do not prevent suit.

5: c. Abandonment occurs when aid or treatment is begun and then discontinued before the patient is turned over to another equally or better trained health professional.

6: c. Only a medical examiner or a physician has the legal authority to pronounce a patient dead. The other choices are all appropriate functions for the EMT to perform.

7: d. All of these actions will tend to ease a patient's anxiety and establish you as a professional.

Practical Applications

Consider how you would act, and why, in the following situations.

1. You are called to a home by an anxious wife. The husband tells you that he suffered chest pains but they're gone now, so it was probably just gas. She insists that you take him to the hospital, but he refuses.

2. The door to a home is opened when you knock, and a woman tells you "Yes, I did call you but I've changed my mind"; says "Thank you," and closes the door.

3. You are at a home treating a middle aged male patient when you hear over your radio that there has been a motor vehicle accident near by.

4. A child riding her bicycle alone has been hit by a car. She is conscious when you get there. The person that called you says the child does not live in the neighborhood.

5. You pull your ambulance up to the emergency department. You and your partner assist the patient into a chair, but speak to no hospital staff. Your partner suggests you "get going, and hurry back to base."

6. You are alone and see a motor vehicle accident on a highway. Neither the police nor ambulance personnel have arrived.

7. You are treating a victim of a motor vehicle accident when a man approaches and states that he is a doctor. He tells you to follow a course of treatment that you do not think is appropriate.

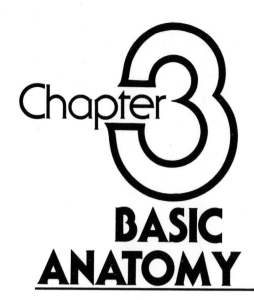

Chapter 3

BASIC ANATOMY

Comprehensive Questions

1. Why is it important for the EMT to learn and use standard anatomical terms?

2. Why is it necessary to know the relationship between external body landmarks and internal structures and organs?

3. What are the major sections of the body? Name the structures and organs that are found in each.

Reference Data

ANATOMICAL TERMINOLOGY

1. When referring to a point on or in the body it is assumed that the body is being viewed from the front, standing erect, with arms at the sides and palms facing forward.

2. **Left** and **right** refer to the *patient's* left and right.

3. **Anterior** refers to the front surface of the body, or, in relating two positions, to the point toward the front.

4. **Posterior** refers to the back surface of the body, or, in relating two points, to the point toward the back.

5. **Midline** refers to an imaginary vertical line running from the mid-forehead through the nose, the umbilicus, and straight to the ground.

6. **Medial** refers to a surface facing the midline.

7. **Lateral** refers to a surface facing away from the midline.

8. **Proximal** refers to a position on an extremity nearer the trunk, to a position on the trunk nearer the midline, or to a position nearer to a named reference point.

9. **Distal** refers to a position on an extremity farther from the trunk, to a position on the trunk farther from the midline, or to a position farther from a named reference point.

10. **Superior** refers to a position toward the head.

11. **Inferior** refers to a position toward the feet.

Review Questions

Select the correct answer for each of the following questions. There is only *one* correct answer for each.

1. Anatomically, the term "superior" means located:
    a. above.
    b. in front.
    c. in back.
    d. below.

2. The term "thorax" refers to the:
    a. brain case.
    b. back of the neck.
    c. pelvic cavity.
    d. chest.

3. The term "anterior" refers to the:
    a. front surface of the body.
    b. rear surface of the body.
    c. surface toward the midline.
    d. surface away from the midline.

4. The anatomical term for the "Adam's apple" is the:
    a. pharynx.
    b. larynx.
    c. esophagus.
    d. epiglottis.

5. The superior boundary of the abdomen is the:
    a. diaphragm.
    b. pelvic girdle.
    c. posterior wall.
    d. anterior wall.

6. The "medial aspect" of a bone is that portion of the bone:
    a. toward the midline of the body.
    b. away from the midline of the body.
    c. nearer to the back.
    d. nearer a free end.

7. The inferior boundary of the thorax is the:
    a. diaphragm.
    b. pelvic girdle.
    c. midline.
    d. abdomen.

8. Anatomically, the term "distal" means:
    a. toward the midline of the body.
    b. away from the midline of the body.
    c. nearer the trunk.
    d. on the front surface.

9. The skin:
    a. is the largest organ of the body.
    b. regulates heat.
    c. protects against infection.
    d. all of the above.

10. The "inferior aspect" of an organ is that portion of the organ:
    a. toward the head of the body.
    b. toward the feet of the body.
    c. toward the midline of the body.
    d. away from the midline of the body.

11. The bone which forms the lower jaw is the:
    a. mastoid.
    b. maxilla.
    c. mandible.
    d. cranium.

12. In the neck, the esophagus lies:
    a. anterior to the trachea.
    b. posterior to the cervical vertebrae.
    c. posterior to the trachea.
    d. within the cricoid cartilage.

13. The flap of tissue that acts to prevent food or liquid from entering the lungs is called the:
    a. trachea.
    b. bronchus.
    c. epiglottis.
    d. larynx.

14. Two passageways extend downward from the throat. The tube that carries air to the lungs is called the:
    a. trachea.
    b. bronchus.
    c. larynx.
    d. esophagus.

15. The major organs of the thorax include the:
    a. esophagus, trachea, and larynx.
    b. heart, lungs, and spleen.
    c. heart, lungs, and esophagus.
    d. stomach, lungs, and liver.

16. The costal arch is made up of:
    a. the clavicle and the sternum.
    b. the costal cartilage of the fifth through tenth ribs.
    c. the costal cartilage of the first through fifth ribs.
    d. the two sets of floating ribs.

17. The heart lies in the chest:
    a. superior to the lungs.
    b. at the level of the seventh to the tenth ribs.
    c. completely to the right of the midline.
    d. immediately posterior to the sternum.

18. The stomach lies in what quadrant of the abdomen?
    a. Right upper.
    b. Left upper.
    c. Right lower.
    d. Left lower.

19. The pelvis is composed of the sacrum and the innominate bone.
    The innominate bone is a fusion of:
    a. the 5 lumbar vertebrae.
    b. the greater and the lesser trochanters.
    c. the ilium, the ischium, and the pubis.
    d. the femur and the pubis.

20. The major artery which supplies blood to the lower extremity is
    the:
    a. carotid.
    b. femoral.
    c. subclavian.
    d. brachial.

Answers to Review Questions

1: a. The term "superior" refers to a point or structure above another: *e.g.,* the humerus is superior to the radius and ulna.

2: d. The thorax is the chest area.

3: a. The term "anterior" refers to the front surface of the body.

4: b. The larynx may protrude from the anterior surface of the neck. It is known as the "Adam's apple."

5: a. The diaphragm is the superior boundary of the abdomen.

6: a. The term "medial" means toward the midline.

7: a. The diaphragm is the inferior boundary of the thorax. It separates the thorax from the abdomen.

8: b. "Distal" refers to a point farther away from the midline, or another reference point. Proximal refers to a nearer point.

9: d. All of these are true of the skin.

10: b. The term "inferior" refers to the undersurface of an organ, or to an organ or structure lying below another.

11: c. The mandible is the bone forming the lower jaw.

12: c. The esophagus lies posterior to, or behind, the trachea.

13: c. The epiglottis closes over the opening to the trachea whenever food or liquid is present in the pharynx.

14: a. Air passes from the outside through the trachea to the lungs.

15: c. The heart, lungs, and esophagus are major organs located in the thorax.

16: b. The costal arch is formed by the costal cartilage of the fifth through the tenth ribs.

17: d. The heart lies immediately posterior to the sternum.

18: b. The stomach lies in the left upper quadrant of the abdomen, protected by the lower portion of the left rib cage.

19: c. The innominate bone is a fusion of the ilium, ischium, and pubis. It connects with the sacrum to form the ring of bone called the pelvis.

20: b. The femoral artery supplies blood to the lower extremity.

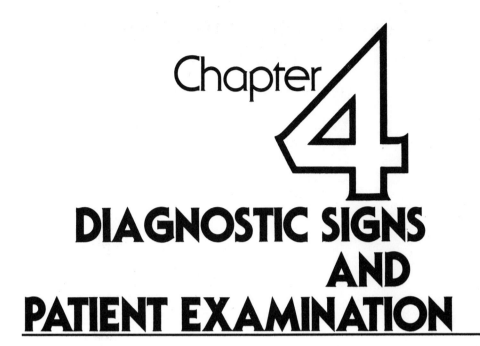

Chapter 4

DIAGNOSTIC SIGNS
AND
PATIENT EXAMINATION

Comprehensive Questions

1. What are the diagnostic signs? Describe what information each gives you.

2. What are the normal vital sign ranges for adults? for children? for infants?

3. Why are mechanism of injury and the patient's history considered diagnostic indicators?

4. Why is the taking of vital signs and the checking of other key indicators important in treating a sick or injured patient?

5. Explain how each of the following gives you information about the adequacy of perfusion: taking the pulse, noting the skin color and temperature, noting the difference between central and distal circulation, using a sphygmomanometer.

6. What diagnostic signs help you evaluate a patient's ventilation?

7. Describe in sequence and detail how you would examine an unconscious patient to determine his condition and the extent of his injuries. Do the same for a conscious patient.

Performance Skills

1. Evaluate and record the rate and quality of a patient's respiration.

2. Evaluate and record the rate and quality of a patient's pulse.

3. Evaluate and record a patient's blood pressure by auscultation.

4. Evaluate and record a patient's blood pressure by palpation.

5. Evaluate and record the temperature and color of a patient's skin.

6. Evaluate and record a patient's pupillary reactions.

7. Evaluate a patient's state of consciousness.

8. Evaluate a conscious patient's neurological status.

9. Evaluate an unconscious patient's neurological status.

10. Examine the patient's entire body in a methodical way to discover evidence of any problem or injury.

11. Perform the primary survey for life-threatening conditions.

Reference Data

PATIENT EXAMINATION

1. **Primary Survey**
   a. Is the patient or the EMT in a dangerous environment?
   b. Is the patient conscious or unconscious?
   c. Does the patient have spontaneous ventilation?
   d. Does the patient have spontaneous circulation?
   e. Does the patient have major external bleeding?

2. **Primary Observation**
   a. Does the patient's general appearance indicate a life-threatening systemic condition?

3. **Basic Signs**
   The basic diagnostic signs and symptoms include:
   a. respiration
   b. pulse
   c. blood pressure
   d. skin temperature
   e. skin color
   f. status and reactiveness of pupils
   g. state of consciousness
   h. reaction to pain
   i. ability to move
   j. history of the incident (mechanism of injury)
   k. medical history

4. **Full Body Survey**
   Is there any injury, tenderness, or deformity to the:
   a. sternum, ribs, chest, or small of the back?
   b. abdomen?
   c. pelvis, genitalia, or buttocks?
   d. head or maxillofacial area?
   e. cervical area?
   f. clavicle or scapula?
   g. arms?
   h. legs?

PATIENT NORMS

1. **Rate of Respiration**
   Rate is given as the number of ventilations per minute.
   Adults: average: 16 to 18 per minute.
   normal range: 12 to 20 per minute.

Children:

average: 20 to 24 per minute.

normal range: 18 to 30 per minute.

Infants:

average: 40 per minute.

normal range: 30 to 50 per minute.

2. **Pulse Rate**

The rate is given as the number of beats per minute.

Adults:

normal range: 60 to 100 per minute.

Children:

normal range: 80 to 110 per minute.

Infants:

normal range: 80 to 160 per minute.

Tachycardia: a pulse rate of 100 per minute or above in an adult.

Bradycardia: a pulse rate of 60 per minute or below in an adult.

3.

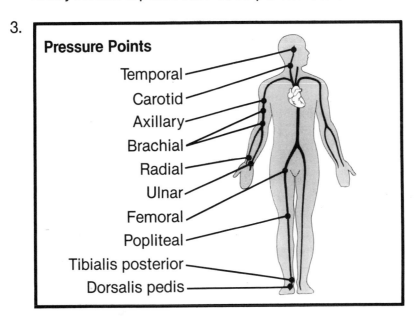

Pressure Points

Temporal
Carotid
Axillary
Brachial
Radial
Ulnar
Femoral
Popliteal
Tibialis posterior
Dorsalis pedis

4. **Blood Pressure**

Blood pressure is measured in millimeters of mercury (mm Hg).

a. **Systolic** pressure is that which exists during the contractions of the heart.

b. **Diastolic** pressure is that which exists while the heart relaxes.

c. BP is reported as systolic "over" diastolic: $\frac{\text{systolic}}{\text{diastolic}}$

Adult males:

normal range: $\dfrac{90 \text{ to } 140}{60 \text{ to } 90}$

Adult females:

normal range: $\dfrac{80 \text{ to } 140}{60 \text{ to } 90}$

Children:

normal range: systolic of 80 plus the patient's age.

Infants:

normal range: systolic of 70 to 90.

    d. Hypertension—a systolic value of 150 mm Hg in an adult.

    e. Hypotension—a systolic value of 90 mm Hg or below in an adult.

Review Questions

Select the correct answer for each of the following questions. There is only *one* correct answer for each.

1. The *normal* heart rate of an average adult is:
    a. 12 to 16 beats per minute.
    b. approximately 20 beats per minute.
    c. 60 to 100 beats per minute.
    d. approximately 100 beats plus the adult's age.

2. The *normal* respiratory rate of an average adult is:
    a. 6 to 12 ventilations per minute.
    b. 16 to 18 ventilations per minute.
    c. 22 to 26 ventilations per minute.
    d. 20 to 30 ventilations per minute.

3. A patient's pulse quality can be affected by:
    a. a loss of blood volume.
    b. dilation of the vessels without blood loss.
    c. malfunctioning of the heart.
    d. all of the above.

4. To evaluate a patient's skin temperature, the EMT should use:
    a. the palm of his hand.
    b. his index and middle fingers.
    c. the back of his hand.
    d. the tips of his fingers.

5. When evaluating a patient's pulse, you are:
    a. counting the waves of blood which the heart sends through an artery.
    b. feeling the swelling of a vein as each wave of blood passes back to the heart.
    c. noting the heart beats in the column of blood in a large vein.
    d. feeling the vibration of the heart muscles as they push the blood through the blood vessels.

6. In dark-skinned people, cyanosis may be seen by observing the:
    a. knuckles.
    b. abdomen.
    c. tongue and nail beds.
    d. ear lobes.

7. The assessment of a patient's eyes includes:
    a. reactivity of the pupils.
    b. ability of the eyes to focus.
    c. ability of the eyes to track properly.
    d. all of the above.

8. An adult male should be considered in a life-threatening condition if his systolic pressure is below:
   a. 150.
   b. 125.
   c. 100.
   d. 90.

9. When you are taking a patient's blood pressure by auscultation, you determine the systolic pressure by:
   a. noting the point on the gauge at which the sound disappears or changes in quality.
   b. noting the point on the gauge at which the needle starts moving.
   c. noting the point on the gauge at which you first hear a strong sound.
   d. inflating the bulb of the sphygmomanometer until it reaches 200 mm Hg.

10. The EMT can palpate the radial pulse:
    a. at the wrist proximal to the thumb.
    b. in the groin.
    c. in the neck below the angle of the jaw.
    d. at the inner aspect of the elbow.

11. A "bounding" pulse is:
    a. normal.
    b. stronger than normal.
    c. weaker than normal.
    d. barely palpable.

12. The absence of a pulse in a specific artery may mean that:
    a. that artery is blocked.
    b. that artery is injured.
    c. the heart has stopped functioning.
    d. all of the above.

13. A pulse is most readily felt at points:
    a. where the artery is close to the skin.
    b. where the artery is located directly over a bone.
    c. where the artery is located both close to the skin and directly over a bone.
    d. none of the above. (A pulse can easily be detected anywhere in the body.)

14. The rate of respiration may vary as a result of a patient's:
    a. physical condition.
    b. apprehension.
    c. physical activity.
    d. all of the above.

15. While taking a blood pressure on a patient, the EMT should remember that *normal* systolic pressure in an adult male is estimated to be:
    a. 90 plus the patient's age, not to exceed 140.
    b. 95 plus the patient's age, not to exceed 140.
    c. 100 plus the patient's age, not to exceed 140.
    d. 105 plus the patient's age, not to exceed 140.

16. The carotid pulse:
    a. can be found on the inner aspect of the arm.
    b. lies lateral to the larynx.
    c. is on the thumb side of the wrist.
    d. is located in the groin of each thigh.

17. When evaluating a patient's respiration, the EMT should observe and record:
    a. rate and rhythm.
    b. rate and degree of chest movement.
    c. rhythm and degree of chest movement.
    d. rate, rhythm, and degree of chest movement.

18. You would expect the systolic pressure of an adult female to be:
    a. 65 to 90 mm Hg.
    b. 100 plus the patient's age.
    c. 8 to 10 mm Hg lower than that of a male of the same age and physical condition.
    d. 10 to 20 mm Hg higher than that of a male of the same age and physical condition.

19. Which of the following is not required when taking a patient's BP by palpation?
    a. An aneroid sphygmomanometer.
    b. A mercurial sphygmomanometer.
    c. A stethoscope.
    d. All are required.

20. Labored or difficult breathing is called:
    a. hyperpnea.
    b. dyspnea.
    c. apnea.
    d. orthopnea.

21. If you have difficulty in obtaining a patient's blood pressure:
    a. tape the diaphragm bell in the proper position.
    b. attempt to palpate the brachial pulse.
    c. have the patient raise his arm before inflating the cuff again.
    d. all of the above.

22. Change in blood pressure indicates change in:
    a. blood volume.
    b. the elasticity of the vessels.
    c. the ability of the heart to pump.
    d. any or all of these.

23. When taking a patient's blood pressure by palpation, as the cuff is deflated, the EMT should note and record the value on the gauge:
    a. when the needle begins to move.
    b. when he first hears a pulse sound.
    c. when the pulse sounds disappear.
    d. when the patient's radial pulse is felt.

24. The normal pulse rate of an average adult is found within the range of:
    a. 15 to 90 per minute.
    b. 40 to 60 per minute.
    c. 60 to 100 per minute.
    d. 80 to 120 per minute.

25. When reporting a patient's blood pressure taken by palpation, which value is omitted?
    a. Systolic.
    b. Diastolic.

Answers to Review Questions

1: c. The normal heart rate of an average adult is usually within the range of 60 to 100 beats per minute.

2: b. The normal respiratory rate of an average adult is usually within the range of 16 to 18 ventilations per minute.

3: d. All of these factors can affect a patient's pulse quality.

4: c. The EMT should use the back of his hand since the palm is less sensitive.

5: a. The pulse is the wave or surge of blood moving through an artery due to the contraction of the heart.

6: c. The tongue and nail beds of dark-skinned people will show a bluish tint if cyanosis is present.

7: d. All of the choices listed should be tested when assessing a patient's eyes.

8: d. While normal systolic pressure will vary from patient to patient, 90 mm Hg indicates life-threat, particularly if 90 is a lower value than that found in a previous reading.

9: c. The point at which you first hear the sound of a pulse wave is the patient's systolic pressure. The diastolic pressure is noted when the sound disappears.

10: a. The radial pulse is palpated at the wrist, proximal to the thumb.

11: b. A "bounding" pulse is stronger than normal.

12: d. Any of the factors listed may be responsible for the absence of a pulse.

13: c. A pulse is most readily palpated where an artery is both close to the skin and over a bone.

14: d. All the factors listed can affect a patient's respiratory rate.

15: c. The rule of thumb for normal systolic pressure in the adult male is 100 plus the patient's age, not to exceed 140.

16: b. The carotid arteries are lateral to the larynx.

17: d. Rate, rhythm, and degree of chest movement should all be assessed when evaluating respiration.

18: c. An average female's blood pressure is 8 to 10 mm Hg lower than that of a comparable male.

19: c. A stethoscope is not needed to take a blood pressure by palpation.

20: b. The term *dyspnea* describes air hunger resulting in difficult or labored breathing.

21: d. All of these are "trouble-shooting" tips that are helpful in obtaining a blood pressure.

22: d. All of these factors can affect or cause changes in a patient's blood pressure.

23: d. The point at which the radial pulse is felt indicates the value when using the palpation method.

24: c. The normal adult pulse range is between 60 and 100 beats per minute.

25: b. The diastolic value is not available by the palpation method.

Chapter 5

THE RESPIRATORY AND CIRCULATORY SYSTEMS

Comprehensive Questions

1. Draw and label a model of the structures and organs that make up the respiratory (ventilatory) system.

2. Explain the muscular and mechanical processes by which ventilation takes place.

3. Draw and label a model of the structures and organs that make up the circulatory system.

4. Describe the mechanical process by which blood is circulated to the cells of the body.

5. Explain how the ventilatory and circulatory systems work together to bring oxygen to the body cells and expel carbon dioxide.

6. Describe the exchange of gases at the cellular level.

7. How does a body cell that is not immediately adjacent to a capillary exchange oxygen and carbon dioxide?

8. Describe the physiological differences in the structure of arteries, veins, and capillaries.

9. Draw a diagram of the heart. Explain how it functions.

10. Describe the process by which the heart cells are oxygenated.

11. Describe the difference between the pulmonary circulation and the systemic circulation.

12. List the major components of blood and the functions each serves.

13. The respiratory and circulatory systems are constantly self-adjusting. Explain the processes which cause:
    a. change in the rate and depth of ventilations.
    b. change in the rate and strength of the heartbeat.
    c. change in the diameter of blood vessels.

Reference Data

RESPIRATORY SYSTEM

1. **Respiration** is the process whereby oxygen and carbon dioxide are exchanged between the atmosphere and the cells of the body. The process includes the following four basic functions.
   a. The exchange of gases between the atmosphere and the lungs.
   b. The exchange of gases between the lungs and the blood.
   c. The transportation of the gases from the lungs to the body cells and from the body cells to the lungs.
   d. The exchange of gases between the blood and the body cells.

2. The **major structures** of the respiratory system include:
   a. the nose and mouth
   b. the pharynx
   c. the larynx
   d. the trachea
   e. bronchi and bronchioles
   f. the lungs (including the capillary network surrounding the alveoli)

3.
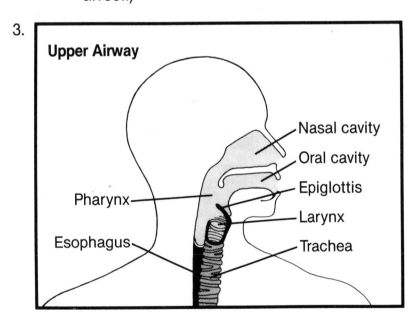

Upper Airway

Nasal cavity
Oral cavity
Epiglottis
Pharynx
Larynx
Esophagus
Trachea

4. The **lung capacity** of the average adult male is about 6 quarts (6 liters).

5. The amount of air exchanged with each ventilation, called the **tidal volume,** is about one pint (500 ml).

6. The amount of air that remains in the lungs, the **residual volume,** is therefore about 5 and 1/2 quarts (5 and 1/2 liters).

7. The average **rate of respiration** for an adult is about 16 to 18 ventilations per minute. Respiratory rate is affected by exercise, rest, physical condition, age, disease, trauma, and emotional state.

8. **Inspired air** contains approximately 20 percent oxygen.

9. **Expired air** contains approximately 16 percent oxygen, and 4 percent carbon dioxide.

CIRCULATORY SYSTEM

1. **Circulation** is the movement of blood through the vessels of the body and the heart.

2. The **major structures** of the circulatory system include:
   a. the heart
   b. the arteries and arterioles
   c. the veins and the venules
   d. the capillaries
   e. the blood

3.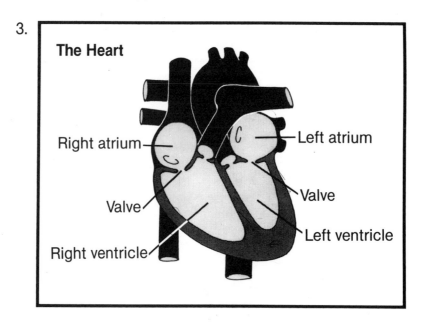

The Heart

Right atrium

Left atrium

Valve

Valve

Right ventricle

Left ventricle

4. **Pulmonary circulation:** the right side of the heart pumps deoxygenated blood to the lungs via the pulmonary artery (the only artery that carries deoxygenated blood), and oxygenated blood from the lungs back to the left side of the heart via the pulmonary vein (the only vein that carries oxygenated blood).

5. **Systemic circulation:** the left side of the heart pumps oxygenated blood to cells throughout the body via the aorta and its branches, and deoxygenated blood back to the right side of the heart.

6. Some **major arteries** of the circulatory system include:
   a. the aorta
   b. the coronary arteries
   c. the right and left common **carotid arteries,** which carry blood to the head and the brain
   d. the **brachial arteries** and their subdivisions, which carry blood to the arms
   e. the **femoral arteries** and their subdivisions, which carry blood to the legs

7. The **quantity of blood** in the circulatory system of an average adult is 6 liters. Children have proportionately less; a newborn has about 300 ml.

8. The **major components of blood** are:
   a. **plasma.** This is the liquid portion of the blood in which the solid components are suspended.
   b. **erythrocytes** (red blood cells). These cells contain hemoglobin, a chemical that combines rapidly with oxygen and carries it to the body cells.
   c. **leukocytes** (white blood cells). These cells fight infection by engulfing foreign particles or by forming antibodies.
   d. **platelets.** These cells allow the blood to clot by disintegrating and combining with proteins in the plasma.

Review Questions

Select the correct answer for each of the following questions. There is only *one* correct answer for each.

1. When the chest muscles contract and pull the rib cage outward, and the diaphragm moves downward, the lungs expand and air rushes in. This phase of breathing is known as:
   a. respiration.
   b. expiration.
   c. inspiration.
   d. ventilation.

2. The flap of tissue that prevents food or liquid from entering the lungs is called the:
   a. trachea.
   b. bronchus.
   c. epiglottis.
   d. larynx.

3. Two passageways extend downward from the throat to the lungs and stomach, respectively. The tube that carries air to the lungs is called the:
   a. trachea.
   b. bronchus.
   c. larynx.
   d. esophagus.

4. In the lungs, oxygen and carbon dioxide are exchanged through the walls of the:
   a. pulmonary arteries.
   b. pulmonary veins.
   c. pulmonary capillaries.
   d. pulmonary venules.

5. An average adult at rest moves approximately 500 ml of air with each breath. This volume is called the:
   a. residual volume.
   b. residual capacity.
   c. tidal volume.
   d. reserve volume.

6. Two passageways extend from the throat through the neck. The tube that carries ingested food from the mouth to the stomach is called the:
   a. trachea.
   b. esophagus.
   c. larynx.
   d. epiglottis.

7. Blood goes to the lungs for oxygenation from which chamber?
   a. Left ventricle.
   b. Left atrium.
   c. Right ventricle.
   d. Right atrium.

8. Blood is carried away from the heart in vessels called:
   a. arteries.
   b. veins.
   c. capillaries.
   d. venules.

9. The air we *inhale* contains about:
   a. 16 percent oxygen.
   b. 20 percent oxygen.
   c. 40 percent oxygen.
   d. 80 percent oxygen.

10. The air we *exhale* contains about:
   a. 16 percent oxygen.
   b. 20 percent oxygen.
   c. 40 percent oxygen.
   d. 80 percent oxygen.

11. The rate and depth of breathing are regulated by:
   a. the brain.
   b. the diaphragm.
   c. the muscles of the ribs.
   d. the spinal cord.

12. During exhalation, the muscles of the ribs and diaphragm:
   a. contract.
   b. stretch.
   c. relax.
   d. none of the above.

13. During inhalation, the muscles of the ribs and diaphragm:
   a. contract.
   b. expand.
   c. relax.
   d. none of the above.

14. The pleural space is:
   a. a potential space, normally without air or fluid.
   b. the area in the lungs where oxygen exchange takes place.
   c. the space between the lungs.
   d. the membrane important in the mechanism of respiration.

15. Breathing is usually controlled by the brain's sensitivity to the blood's level of:
    a. oxygen.
    b. carbon dioxide.
    c. carbon monoxide.
    d. nitrogen.

16. The principal artery of the body is the:
    a. radial.
    b. femoral.
    c. aorta.
    d. brachial.

17. The smooth, glistening, membranous sac that surrounds each lung is called the:
    a. visceral pleura.
    b. diaphragm.
    c. mesentery.
    d. peritoneum.

18. Blood functions to:
    a. regulate body temperature.
    b. transport oxygen and nutrients.
    c. transport carbon dioxide and other wastes.
    d. all of the above.

19. Blood is carried toward the heart in vessels called:
    a. arteries.
    b. veins.
    c. capillaries.
    d. arterioles.

20. The pulmonary circulation functions primarily to:
    a. transport oxygenated blood throughout the body and deoxygenated blood to the heart.
    b. transport deoxygenated blood to the lungs and oxygenated blood to the heart.
    c. transport oxygenated blood to the body cells.
    d. transport deoxygenated blood to the heart.

21. The systemic circulation functions primarily to:
    a. transport oxygenated blood throughout the body and deoxygenated blood back to the heart.
    b. transport deoxygenated blood to the lungs and oxygenated blood to the heart.
    c. transport oxygenated blood from the lungs to the heart.
    d. transport deoxygenated blood from the heart to the lungs.

22. While blood volume varies with body size and weight, a rule of thumb is that an average adult male has:
    a. 8 pints (4 liters) of blood.
    b. 10 pints (5 liters) of blood.
    c. 12 pints (6 liters) of blood.
    d. 15 pints (8 liters) of blood.

23. The solid components of blood that are essential to respiration are the:
    a. erythrocytes (red blood cells).
    b. leukocytes (white blood cells).
    c. platelets.
    d. plasma.

24. The solid components of blood that are essential to clotting are the:
    a. erythrocytes (red blood cells).
    b. leukocytes (white blood cells).
    c. platelets.
    d. plasma.

25. The solid components of blood that are active "disease fighters" are the:
    a. erythrocytes (red blood cells).
    b. leukocytes (white blood cells).
    c. platelets.
    d. plasma.

26. What part of the body receives its blood supply from the brachial artery?
    a. Brain.
    b. Myocardium.
    c. Thigh.
    d. Upper arm.

27. The fluid portion of blood is:
    a. erythrocyte.
    b. leukocyte.
    c. platelet.
    d. plasma.

28. Oxygen carried in the blood is exchanged for carbon dioxide and other cellular waste materials through the walls of the:
    a. arteries.
    b. veins.
    c. capillaries.
    d. arterioles.

29. Arteries can constrict or dilate because they are lined with:
   a. elastic tissue.
   b. striated muscle tissue.
   c. smooth muscle tissue.
   d. voluntary muscles.

30. Veins have special structures to prevent the back flow of blood. These structures are:
   a. valves.
   b. fibrils.
   c. tendrils.
   d. glands.

Answers to Review Questions

1: c. Air rushes in during the inspiratory phase of breathing.

2: c. The epiglottis closes over the trachea when we swallow.

3: a. The trachea carries air to the lungs; the esophagus connects the pharynx and stomach; a bronchus is a branch of the trachea within each lung; and the larynx is the voice box above the trachea.

4: c. Oxygen and carbon dioxide are exchanged through the walls of the pulmonary capillaries. The term pulmonary refers to anything involving or concerning the lungs.

5: c. Tidal volume is the amount of air normally inhaled and exhaled. Residual volume refers to the amount of air that is always present in the lungs.

6: b. The esophagus carries food to the stomach; the trachea carries air to the lungs.

7: c. The right ventricle pumps deoxygenated blood to the lungs through the pulmonary arteries.

8: a. Arteries carry blood *from* the heart; veins carry blood *to* the heart; capillaries connect arterioles and venules; venules are small veins.

9: b. The air we normally breathe contains approximately 20 percent oxygen and 79 percent nitrogen.

10: a. The air we exhale contains approximately 16 percent oxygen, and approximately 4 percent carbon dioxide.

11: a. While all are involved in breathing, the brain controls the rate and depth.

12: c. These muscles relax, the chest cavity becomes smaller, and air moves from the lungs.

13: a. These muscles contract, the chest cavity becomes larger, and air enters due to the lower pressure created.

14: a. The pleural space is a potential space. The visceral and parietal pleurae normally are in contact with each other.

15: b. Breathing is controlled by the level of carbon dioxide in the blood. In some conditions, the part of the brain that senses this fails. The body then uses an alternate system that reacts to the level of oxygen.

16: c. The aorta is the principal artery in the body.

17: a. The visceral pleura surrounds the lungs; the parietal pleura lines the thorax.

18: d. All the items listed are functions of the blood.

19: b. Vessels called veins carry blood to the heart.

20: b. The pulmonary circulation functions to transport deoxygenated blood to the lungs, and oxygenated blood from the lungs to the heart.

21: a. The systemic circulation pumps oxygenated blood from the heart throughout the body and deoxygenated blood to the heart.

22: c. The average adult male has approximately 12 pints of blood.

23: a. Erythrocytes (red blood cells) are essential to respiration. The hemoglobin they contain combines with oxygen and transports it to the body tissues.

24: c. Platelets break apart and their components undergo a series of chemical changes resulting in a blood clot.

25: b. Leukocytes, the white blood cells, fight infection and disease by engulfing foreign particles or by producing chemical agents to neutralize them.

26: d. The brachial arteries and their branches, including the radial and ulnar arteries, bring oxygenated blood to the arms.

27: d. The fluid portion of the blood is plasma. The solid components are suspended within the plasma.

28: c. Gases, as well as nutrients and wastes, are exchanged through the walls of the capillaries.

29: c. The walls of arteries are made up of smooth muscle tissue.

30: a. Valves located within the veins prevent backward flow of the blood.

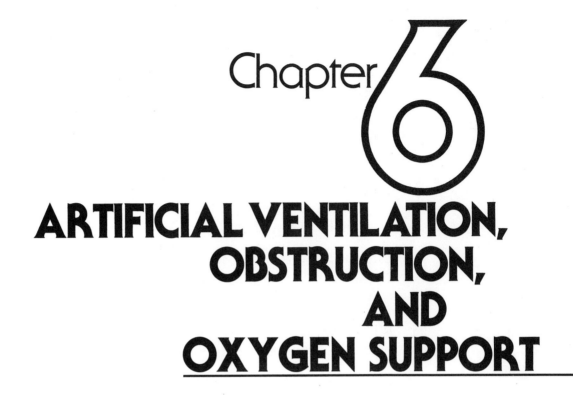

Chapter 6

ARTIFICIAL VENTILATION, OBSTRUCTION, AND OXYGEN SUPPORT

Comprehensive Questions

1. Respiration is normally an effortless, spontaneous process. When this process no longer occurs spontaneously, what is the primary need of the patient? How quickly must treatment be provided?

2. What is artificial ventilation? How is it different from spontaneous respiration?

3. What are the commonly used devices for oxygen-assisted artificial ventilation? Discuss the situations where each might be used and the advantages and disadvantages of each.

4. What is the basic purpose of oxygen support of a patient who is breathing?

5. What are the commonly used devices for oxygen support of a breathing patient? Discuss the situations in which each might be used and the advantages and disadvantages of each.

6. What is the purpose of an oropharyngeal or nasopharyngeal airway? In what situations should one be used? When is their use contraindicated?

7. Explain why abdominal compression is an effective maneuver for clearing an obstructed airway.

Performance Skills

1. Treat a conscious patient with an obstructed airway using a combination of back blows and abdominal compressions.

2. Treat an unconscious patient with an obstructed airway using a combination of back blows and abdominal thrusts.

3. Establish and maintain a patient airway:
   a. by the head-tilt method.
   b. by the jaw-lift method.
   c. by the jaw-thrust method.

4. Assess the need for, and perform, mouth-to-mouth resuscitation on an adult patient.

5. Assess the need for, and perform, mouth-to-mouth resuscitation on an infant.

6. Assess the need for, and perform, mouth-to-nose resuscitation on an adult patient.

7. Assess the need for, and perform, mouth-to-stoma resuscitation.

8. Use portable and on-board suction equipment to assist in managing a patient's airway.

9. Ventilate an unconscious patient with an oxygen-enriched pocket mask.

10. Correctly measure and insert an oropharyngeal airway.

11. Use oxygen-enriched positive pressure equipment (bag-valve-mask and demand-valve resuscitator) to resuscitate a patient.

12. Use oxygen-enriched, positive pressure equipment to support inadequate spontaneous ventilations of an unconscious patient.

13. Provide oxygen support (nasal cannula, simple face mask, pocket mask, mask and bag) to a conscious patient that is breathing spontaneously.

14. Start oxygen and adjust the flow rate.

Reference Data

1. Cells of the nervous system, particularly the brain, begin to die in 4 to 6 minutes when deprived of sufficient oxygen.

2. **Rates for artificial ventilation**
   Adults: 1 ventilation every 5 seconds (12 per minute)
   Children 1 to 8 years (or comparable body size): 1 ventilation every 4 seconds (15 per minute)
   Infants: 1 ventilation every 3 seconds (20 per minute)

3. **Oxygen-assisted ventilation equipment**
   a. Pocket mask can deliver 50 to 55 percent oxygen at 10 liters per minute.
   b. Demand-valve resuscitator (with manual triggering) can deliver 100 percent oxygen.
   c. Bag-valve-mask (without reservoir) can deliver 40 percent oxygen at 12 liters per minute.
   d. Bag-valve-mask with oxygen reservoir can deliver 95 percent oxygen at 12 liters per minute.

4. **Oxygen support equipment**
   a. Nasal cannula can deliver 25 to 40 percent oxygen at 4 to 6 liters per minute. (Used to give low-liter flow.)
   b. Simple face-mask can deliver 50 to 60 percent oxygen at 8 to 12 liters per minute. (Used to give high-liter flow.)
   c. Mask and bag (partial rebreathing) can deliver 35 to 60 percent oxygen at 6 to 10 liters per minute.
   d. Mask and bag (non-rebreathing) can deliver 90 percent oxygen at 10 to 12 liters per minute.

Review Questions

Select the correct answer for each of the following questions. There is only *one* correct answer for each.

1. When performing mouth-to-mouth resuscitation, the victim's dentures should be:
    a. removed, because they contain bacteria.
    b. left in, unless loose, because they facilitate making an airtight seal.
    c. removed, because they frequently obstruct the airway.
    d. left in, so they are not lost.

2. When resuscitating an adult patient with the mouth-to-mouth technique, you should provide one breath:
    a. every second, or 60 times per minute.
    b. every 2 seconds, or 30 times per minute.
    c. as often as you can.
    d. every 5 seconds, or 12 times per minute.

3. Which of the following can cause airway obstruction in a patient under the influence of alcohol or other drugs which depress the central nervous system?
    a. May become nauseated and aspirate vomitus.
    b. May not have autonomic reflex to protect the airway from blockage.
    c. May not respond normally to neck flexion.
    d. All of the above.

4. Which of the following must be done when performing mouth-to-stoma resuscitation?
    a. Hyperextend the head.
    b. Ventilate through the nose.
    c. Place mouth directly on stoma, rather than on mouth of the victim.
    d. Extend the patient's head.

5. When using an "S" tube, pocket mask, or other mouth-to-face breathing apparatus on a non-breathing adult patient, you should provide:
    a. half-sized breaths.
    b. regular-sized breaths.
    c. double-sized breaths.
    d. breaths 4 times the normal size.

6. Oxygen can be dangerous because it:
    a. is combustible.
    b. explodes.
    c. supports combustion.
    d. all of these.

7. The most common problem experienced when using a bag mask to administer supplementary oxygen is:
   a. failure to provide a sufficient amount of air.
   b. over-inflation of the patient's lungs.
   c. failure to maintain the proper rate of ventilation.
   d. failure to maintain an adequate seal around the patient's nose and mouth.

8. A patient has a bolus of food which is completely obstructing the airway. To prevent neurological damage it must be dislodged within:
   a. 30 seconds to 1 minute.
   b. 1 to 2 minutes.
   c. 4 to 6 minutes.
   d. 10 minutes.

9. If there is no pulse in either carotid artery, the patient is a victim of:
   a. cardiac arrest.
   b. dyspnea.
   c. CVA.
   d. chronic obstructive lung disease.

10. Exhaled air contains what percentage of oxygen?
    a. 10 percent.
    b. 16 percent.
    c. 21 percent.
    d. 80 percent.

11. You can determine whether an unconscious victim is breathing by:
    a. determining his blood pressure by auscultation.
    b. checking his lips and nail beds for cyanosis.
    c. checking his pulse for rate, rhythm, and quality.
    d. listening, feeling, and looking for signs of air exchange and chest movement.

12. How many breaths per minute should be provided when ventilating an adult laryngectomy patient?
    a. 60.
    b. 30.
    c. 20.
    d. 12.

13. The opening in the neck of a person who has undergone a laryngectomy is called a:
    a. tracheotomy.
    b. stomata.
    c. stoma.
    d. tracheostomy.

14. Having the nose firmly pinched and the head extended, you blow through the mouth and there is no obstruction, but no chest rise. You should:
    a. reposition the head and try again.
    b. proceed to dislodge the obstruction.
    c. check the neck for a stoma.
    d. discontinue life saving attempts.

15. A patient is lying on the ground with no respiration, a weak pulse, and constricted pupils. Which of the following should you do first?
    a. Begin artificial respiration.
    b. Start CPR.
    c. Call for an ambulance.
    d. Ask if anyone knows what happened to this person.

16. After you have established an airway and hyperinflated the non-breathing patient, you should:
    a. go on to regular artificial ventilation.
    b. palpate the carotid arteries to ascertain if spontaneous circulation exists.
    c. give a precordial thump.
    d. treat for shock.

17. You should blow into an arrested patient's lungs:
    a. as hard as you can.
    b. until his abdomen rises.
    c. enough to cause the chest to rise.
    d. until the victim's color improves.

18. Opening the airway for a patient with a head injury differs from the usual technique in that:
    a. the mouth is not swept clear at first.
    b. the head injury is given priority over airway maintenance.
    c. the neck is not hyperextended.
    d. the jaw is not lifted.

19. When maintaining oxygen cylinders, which of the following should *never* be done?
    a. Store cylinders in a cool place.
    b. Apply grease to the valve every month.
    c. Store in upright position in the rack.
    d. Open the valve when the cylinder is empty.

20. Each breath blown during mouth-to-mouth should provide:
    a. 500 ml of air.
    b. 1000 ml of air.
    c. 1500 ml of air.
    d. 2000 ml of air.

21. The simplest technique for opening an airway in most cases is to:
    a. support the neck and tilt the head back.
    b. turn the head to one side.
    c. strike the victim on the back.
    d. wipe out the mouth and throat.

22. At the moment when an unconscious patient has no spontaneous respiration and no spontaneous circulation, the patient is:
    a. DOA—call the medical examiner and coroner.
    b. at the point of biological death.
    c. at the point of clinical death.
    d. legally pronounced dead.

23. When ventilating a patient with a bag-valve-mask, you should squeeze the bag until:
    a. it is empty.
    b. the patient's chest rises.
    c. the patient breathes on his own.
    d. 100 percent oxygen is delivered.

24. After properly squeezing the bag of a bag-valve-mask, you should:
    a. allow it to re-inflate.
    b. squeeze it again.
    c. remove the mask so the patient can exhale.
    d. inflate the bag manually.

25. The curve of an oropharyngeal airway is inserted upside down or sideways at first, then inverted. This is to:
    a. prevent the tongue from being pushed back.
    b. allow the airway to conform to the tongue.
    c. prevent the airway from damaging the teeth.
    d. allow the airway to conform to the shape of the mouth.

26. A patient's nose should be pinched when giving mouth-to-mouth resuscitation to:
    a. maintain even pressure on both lungs.
    b. prevent possible bleeding.
    c. prevent air from escaping when breathing into the patient's mouth.
    d. prevent exhaled air from coming out the patient's nose.

27. Which of the following devices will deliver the highest concentration of oxygen to a patient requiring oxygen support?
    a. Nasal cannula.
    b. Simple face mask.
    c. Non-rebreathing face mask with bag or reservoir.
    d. Venturi mask.

28. You find someone who is apparently unconscious on the floor of his apartment. After determining that neither you nor the patient are in any danger, your first step is to:
    a. feel for a pulse.
    b. position the head.
    c. determine responsiveness.
    d. check the pupils.

29. Which of the following does *not* accurately describe a patient with dyspnea?
    a. Wants to be in a sitting or semi-sitting position.
    b. Is frightened and very anxious.
    c. Is very talkative.
    d. Sucks hard and inefficiently for each breath.

30. When using a demand valve resuscitator or bag-valve-mask to administer supplementary oxygen to an unconscious patient, which of the following should be your first course of action?
    a. Seal the mask to the patient's face.
    b. Elevate the head portion of the ambulance cot.
    c. Place the patient in the coma position.
    d. Make certain an oropharyngeal airway has been inserted.

31. As you attempt to insert an oropharyngeal airway into the throat of an unconscious patient, he begins to gag and retch. You should immediately:
    a. remove it—it may cause this patient to vomit.
    b. remove it and insert a shorter one.
    c. pull it out slightly—it was probably inserted too deeply.
    d. pull it out and reinsert it—it probably wasn't inserted properly the first time.

32. An EMT using a bag-valve-mask resuscitator decides to enrich the oxygen supply. He attaches the oxygen tubing to the mask and adjusts the oxygen flow to:
    a. 4 liters per minute.
    b. 6 liters per minute.
    c. 8 liters per minute.
    d. highest flow rate possible.

33. After inflating the reservoir of an oxygen face mask, the oxygen flow rate should be:
    a. set and maintained at 2 to 4 liters per minute.
    b. adjusted so the reservoir is fully inflated.
    c. set and maintained at 6 to 8 liters per minute.
    d. adjusted so the reservoir neither completely collapses nor is fully inflated.

34. An EMT finds that an accident victim is not breathing. The patient also appears to have an open fracture of his mandible. The EMT should ventilate this patient with:
    a. the chest pressure method.
    b. the back pressure-arm lift method.
    c. the "S" tube.
    d. the mouth-to-nose technique.

35. As a general rule, an EMT should not use suction on an arrested patient for longer than:
    a. 15 seconds.
    b. 10 seconds.
    c. 5 seconds.
    d. 2 seconds.

36. Which of the following is true when opening the airway of a small child?
    a. The child's head should be back as far as possible.
    b. A child's neck is less flexible than an adult's.
    c. Forcing the child's head back too far may result in a collapsed airway.
    d. A child's tongue is more likely to obstruct the airway.

37. When ventilating an infant, the EMT should provide breaths every:
    a. 2 seconds.
    b. 3 seconds.
    c. 4 seconds.
    d. 5 seconds.

38. An advantage of using mouth-to-mouth ventilation with a patient in respiratory arrest is that:
    a. it is the most modern method.
    b. it reduces the amount of air going into the stomach.
    c. it will not produce further injury.
    d. there is better air exchange.

39. Two EMTs find an unconscious, non-breathing patient trapped in a sitting position in a vehicle. Although the victim can be reached, he cannot be removed from the vehicle immediately. The EMTs' first action to aid this patient should be:
    a. get a pry bar and attempt to extricate him from the vehicle in order to get him to a place where he can then be treated safely.
    b. begin ventilating him with a mechanical pressure-cycled resuscitator while the other EMT attempts to extricate him.
    c. support him in an upright position, tilt his head back with his face up, and start ventilating while the other EMT attempts to extricate him.
    d. examine him for any further injuries, since he should not be moved until a thorough evaluation has been made.

40. Excessive volume in infant ventilation may cause:
    a. collapse of the trachea.
    b. rupture of the diaphragm.
    c. pneumothorax.
    d. hemothorax.

41. When you come upon an unconscious victim, you first ascertain that neither you nor the victim are in danger; then ascertain that he is unresponsive. You open the patient's airway properly; then you:
    a. start artificial ventilation.
    b. start CPR.
    c. pinch the nostrils.
    d. look, listen, and feel for evidence of adequate respiration.

42. Which of these procedures occurs first in the proper treatment of an unconscious victim of illness or accident?
    a. Open the airway.
    b. Check for spontaneous circulation.
    c. Administer the abdominal thrust.
    d. Examine the victim for bleeding and fractures.

43. When treating a child, which of the following methods should be used to relieve stomach distention during artificial ventilation?
    a. Hold the child upright and gently pat his back.
    b. Apply heavy pressure on the child's upper abdomen.
    c. Hold the child in an inverted position and strike sharply on his back.
    d. Turn the child's head down or to one side and exert gentle pressure on the child's upper abdomen.

44. After opening the airway and determining that an adult is in respiratory arrest, the EMT should quickly deliver:
    a. 2 double-sized breaths.
    b. 3 double-sized breaths.
    c. 4 double-sized breaths.
    d. 4 regular-sized breaths.

45. The most common causes of airway obstruction in unconscious patients are fluids and:
    a. lower jaw drops down, allowing tongue to obstruct throat.
    b. pieces of food.
    c. debris from injury.
    d. false teeth or bridgework.

46. An unconscious accident victim you are attending exhibits noisy breathing that sounds like snoring. What condition is indicated?
    a. Spasms of the larynx.
    b. Foreign matter in the lungs.
    c. Partial airway obstruction.
    d. Spasms of the bronchi.

47. You are resuscitating an arrested patient with a bag-valve-mask resuscitator. The patient's chest does *not* rise when the bag is squeezed. You should:
    a. squeeze harder on the bag-mask unit.
    b. squeeze easier on the bag-mask unit.
    c. change the mask on the unit.
    d. make a tighter seal with the unit.

48. The best test to determine whether a child needs oxygen is:
    a. if he is more comfortable with it than without it.
    b. his pupillary reaction.
    c. his respiratory rate.
    d. his BP.

49. The mouth-to-stoma technique of artificial ventilation involves the following procedure:
    a. the EMT's mouth is placed directly on the stoma of the patient rather than on his mouth.
    b. the patient is given the same size breaths as a normal breather.
    c. the EMT should watch the patient's chest for elevation.
    d. all of the above.

50. An unconscious patient with a fully obstructed airway should be turned on his side and:
    a. provided with oxygen immediately.
    b. given a series of back blows.
    c. left in the coma position.
    d. provided with an oropharyngeal airway.

51. When delivering abdominal thrusts to a standing patient with an obstructed airway, the EMT's fist should be placed:
    a. on the umbilicus.
    b. on the xiphoid process.
    c. between the umbilicus and the xiphoid process.
    d. on the lower sternum.

52. A simple face mask delivering 8 to 12 liters of oxygen per minute provides approximately:
    a. 15 to 20 percent oxygen.
    b. 50 to 60 percent oxygen.
    c. 80 to 90 percent oxygen.
    d. 100 percent oxygen.

53. A patient is in need of ventilatory assistance if his rate of respiration is:
    a. below 12.
    b. 12 to 14.
    c. 14 to 16.
    d. 16 to 18.

Answers to Review Questions

1: b. Dentures should, if possible, be left in to provide structure to the mouth.

2: d. Provide one breath every 5 seconds, which is 12 per minute.

3: d. All of these factors can cause airway obstruction in an intoxicated patient.

4: c. Mouth-to-stoma resuscitation involves ventilation directly through the stoma into the trachea.

5: c. Regardless of the adjunctive device used, the ventilator should supply double-sized breaths (approximately 1000 ml of air) to the victim.

6: c. While oxygen itself does not burn, it supports combustion.

7: d. The most common problem when using a bag-valve-mask is that the operator does not obtain an adequate seal.

8: c. It must be dislodged in 4 to 6 minutes so that ventilation can be performed to prevent biological death.

9: a. The absence of both carotid pulses indicates cardiac arrest.

10: b. Exhaled air contains 16 percent oxygen, inhaled air contains approximately 20 percent oxygen.

11: d. Determine if a patient has spontaneous ventilation by feeling and listening for air exchange and looking for movement of the chest.

12: d. Ventilate a stoma patient at the same rate as any other adult patient—12 per minute.

13: c. A stoma is the opening in the neck of a laryngectomy patient.

14: a. Reposition the head and try again. Make certain the patient's head is hyperextended and his nose is sealed. If there is still no chest rise, check for a stoma or puncture wound of the chest.

15: a. You should first begin artificial ventilation. Chest compression must *not* be performed on a patient with a palpable pulse.

16: b. After hyperventilating a non-breathing patient, you should palpate the carotid arteries to determine if spontaneous circulation exists.

17: c. You should blow into an arrested patient's lungs with enough force to cause his chest to rise.

18: c. Perform the jaw thrust to open the airway of a patient with a head injury. Since there may also be a cervical injury, the neck must not be hyperextended.

19: b. All these items are good practice when handling and using oxygen except *b*. Grease, or any lubricant, must *never* be applied to the valves.

20: b. Artificial ventilation should provide 1000 ml of air; hence the expression "double-sized breath."

21: a. Tilting the head back causes the trachea to open and the esophagus to close; it is the simplest way to open a patient's airway.

22: c. Clinical death occurs when both spontaneous ventilation and circulation cease.

23: b. You should squeeze the bag of a bag-valve-mask until the patient's chest rises.

24: a. After squeezing the bag of a bag-valve-mask, you should release it and allow it to re-inflate.

25: a. An oropharyngeal airway is inserted upside down or sideways, then inverted so as not to push the tongue back.

26: c. A patient's nose is pinched during ventilation to prevent air from escaping through it.

27: c. A non-rebreathing face mask with a reservoir bag attached will deliver 60 to 100 percent oxygen. A nasal cannula will deliver approximately 40 percent, a simple face mask can deliver approximately 60 percent, and a venturi (according to its design) delivers 24, 28, or 35 percent.

28: c. After ascertaining that neither you nor the patient are in any danger, you should determine if the patient is responsive.

29: c. All of these conditions describe a patient with dyspnea except *c*. A dyspnea patient is not talkative due to respiratory difficulty or air hunger.

30: d. An oropharyngeal airway should be inserted first to prevent the patient's tongue from blocking the airway.

31: a. An oropharyngeal airway must be removed if the patient gags or makes any effort to fight it. This will reduce the possibility of vomiting and aspiration of the vomitus.

32: d. The oxygen flow rate should be set at the highest flow rate possible to ensure highest concentration possible.

33: d. When using a face mask with a reservoir attached, the flow rate should be adjusted so that the bag neither fully inflates nor collapses as the patient breathes.

34: d. Under these circumstances, the EMT should attempt to ventilate with the mouth-to-nose method.

35: c. Since ventilation must be interrupted, suction should not be used for more than 5 seconds.

36: c. Since the cartilage that supports the trachea is not fully developed in an infant or small child, hyperextending the neck may cause the trachea to collapse.

37: b. The rate of artificial ventilation is increased to once every 3 seconds with infants or small children, since their normal respiratory rate is higher than that of adults.

38: b. There is less danger of gastric distention with the mouth-to-mouth method than with oxygen resuscitation devices.

39: c. Since respiration takes priority over other injuries, the EMT should start artificial ventilation immediately, taking care to protect the possibly fractured neck.

40: c. Excessive volume when artifically inflating an infant can cause the lungs to rupture, causing a pneumothorax.

41: d. After determining that the patient is unresponsive and opening his airway, you should feel, listen, and look for spontaneous respiration.

42: a. Opening the airway and determining that the patient has spontaneous respiration is the EMT's first priority.

43: d. To relieve gastric distention in an infant or child, apply gentle pressure on the upper abdomen.

44: c. The EMT should provide 4 double-sized breaths to a patient in respiratory arrest, then palpate the carotid arteries to determine if there is spontaneous circulation.

45: a. Airway obstruction commonly occurs when the patient's jaw drops allowing the tongue to block the airway.

46: c. Snoring sounds indicate a partially obstructed airway.

47: d. The most common failure when attempting to ventilate a patient with bag-valve-mask is not maintaining a tight seal around the patient's nose and mouth.

48: a. If there is a question whether or not oxygen should be administered, the EMT should administer oxygen and then judge the patient's reaction.

49: d. All of the procedures listed should be followed when performing mouth-to-stoma ventilation.

50: b. An unconscious patient with an obstructed airway should be turned on his side and given several sharp blows to the spine between the shoulder blades.

51: c. Abdominal thrusts should be delivered with an upward motion between the umbilicus and the xiphoid process.

52: b. A simple face mask delivers approximately 50 to 60 percent oxygen.

53: a. A patient with a respiratory rate of less than 12 is in need of ventilatory assistance.

Practical Applications

Consider how you would act, and why, in the following situations.

1. A young child in a crib is not breathing. A piece of plastic is found nearby. The infant does not have a pulse and opening the airway does not bring back spontaneous respiration.

2. You respond to a restaurant and find a woman choking on a piece of meat. She is at least 8 months pregnant. She is making choking noises as she tries to breathe, and is clutching her throat.

3. You respond to a call of "a child choking" and find a 14-year-old choking on a piece of candy. He seems to be moving some air with his efforts, but appears cyanotic. A visual inspection of the mouth and throat reveals that the object is just beyond your fingertips.

4. You arrive at the scene to find a construction worker buried to mid-chest in a trench. Other workers are trying to dig him out. He is cyanotic and respirations are 26 and shallow. His pulse is 100. The foreman informs you that it will take at least 10 minutes to clear his chest.

5. You respond to a home to find a young woman whose 2-year-old child has recently died. She is breathing rapidly (rate is 60), feeling dizzy and faint. Her pulse is 120; blood pressure is 120/80. Friends say she was resting comfortably and suddenly woke up in this condition.

6. A 17-year-old girl has just been involved in a family argument. The presenting clinical picture includes dizziness, numbness around the mouth, tingle in the fingertips, and rapid breathing.

7. A 26-year-old male was taking a shower when he suddenly experienced tightness and pain high on the left side of his chest. It progressively grew tighter and he experienced respiratory distress allied with the tightness. Pulse is 110; respirations are 22 and labored; blood pressure is 130/90.

8. You are called to a home by a babysitter to treat a young child who is having breathing difficulty. When you arrive, you find a 6-year-old child with severe dyspnea. The child is very frightened. The babysitter tells you that the child was sleeping, awoke with a hoarse cough, and had trouble breathing. She is not aware of any previous attacks.

9. You respond to a home during a power blackout. A 45-year-old man is found ill in his bedroom which is over the garage. His skin is flushed and you notice that this house is the only one on the block that has electrical power. When you ask the family about the

lights, they tell you they have a gas generator in the garage. The man went to bed early and his wife found him this way. He complains of headache and is short of breath. Pulse is 110; respirations are 30; blood pressure is 130/80.

10. A man is found slumped over his desk. Fellow workers claim he suddenly collapsed. He is making snoring sounds. There is no apparent injury. No medical identification or past medical history is available. Pulse is 90 and strong; respirations are 16 and labored, with snoring; blood pressure is 120/80.

11. You respond for "a man not breathing." You open his airway and don't feel, hear, or see any air exchange. You deliver 4 quick breaths, mouth-to-mouth. His chest doesn't rise, but the stomach inflates, and your breaths meet no resistance.

12. You respond on a hot, dry August day to a park where a young child is in respiratory distress. You can hear wheezing every time the child exhales. The child is very anxious and frightened. The mother states that she has the child's medication in the car. Pulse is rapid; respirations are 30; blood pressure is 120/70.

13. Your patient is an elderly gentlemen who was found at home by his grandchildren. He appears to be in acute respiratory distress. You attempt to obtain a brief history, but cannot understand him because of his severe air hunger. You found him sitting on the edge of a chair, wearing a nasal cannula which is connected to a small oxygen tank. He does not wear any medi-alert identification and no medications are present. Pulse is 120 and bounding; respirations are 30 and noisy; and the patient appears to have to fight to inhale. The muscles of his neck and chest appear to strain with each breath.

14. You respond to a local swimming pool for a diving accident. When you arrive, lifeguards have the victim face up in shallow water and are giving mouth-to-mouth. Witnesses state that the victim struck his head on the end of the diving board. He is unconscious and not breathing, but has a pulse.

15. You are called to render aid to a 25-year-old male who has been knocked unconscious in a fight. When you arrive the patient is not breathing. Bleeding has been severe. Your attempts to deliver adequate ventilation by mouth-to-mouth resuscitation fail because of badly lacerated cheeks and lips.

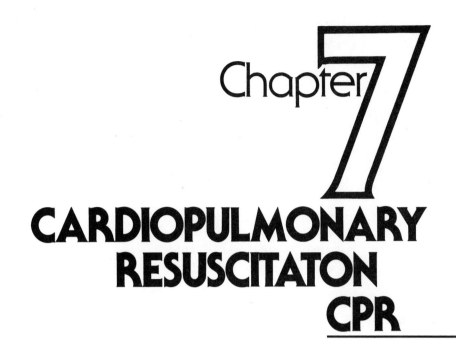

Chapter 7

CARDIOPULMONARY RESUSCITATON CPR

Comprehensive Questions

1. What is the primary purpose of CPR?

2. Differentiate between a patient in need of artificial ventilation and one in need of CPR.

3. Why is it important that CPR not be stopped once it has been started?

4. What is the advantage of oxygen-supported CPR?

5. Why is 2-operator CPR more effective than 1-operator?

6. What are the most common mistakes made in the administration of CPR? What is the physiological result of each of these mistakes.

Performance Skills

1. Assess the need for, and perform, 1-operator CPR:
   a. on an adult.
   b. on a pre-adolescent child.
   c. on an infant.

2. Assess the need for, and perform, 2-operator CPR, including switching positions while maintaining proper compression and ventilation rates:
   a. on an adult.
   b. on a pre-adolescent child.

3. Switch from 1-operator CPR to 2-operator CPR.

4. Determine the effectiveness of CPR while performing it with a second EMT.

5. Switch to oxygen-assisted resuscitation equipment as 2 operators maintain compressions and ventilations.

6. Perform 2-operator CPR as the patient is being moved to the ambulance.

7. Perform 2-operator CPR in a moving ambulance.

8. Perform CPR on:
   a. a stoma patient.
   b. a patient with a puncture wound of the chest.
   c. a patient that has suffered severe hemorrhage.

9. Determine that spontaneous circulation and/or ventilation has returned to a CPR patient.

Reference Data

1. CPR must be started within 4 to 6 minutes after cardiac arrest if it is to prevent irreversible brain damage.

2. The chest compressions performed during CPR are 25 to 33 percent as effective as the normal pumping of the heart.

ONE-OPERATOR CPR

1. **On an adult**
   a. compression rate: 80 per minute
   b. depth of compression: approximately 1½ to 2 inches
   c. compression/ventilation ratio: 15 to 2

2. **On a child**
   a. compression rate: 80 per minute
   b. depth of compression: approximately 1 to 1½ inches
   c. compression/ventilation ratio: 15 to 2 (may use 1 hand only)

3. **On an infant**
   a. compression rate: 80 to 100 per minute
   b. depth of compression: approximately ½ to 1 inch
   c. compression/ventilation ratio: 5 to 1 (no interruption of compressions)

4. **On a newborn**
   a. compression rate: 100 per minute
   b. depth of compression: ½ to ¾ of an inch
   c. compression/ventilation ratio: 5 to 1 (no interruption of compressions)

TWO-OPERATOR CPR

1. **On an adult**
   a. compression rate: 60 per minute
   b. depth of compression: approximately 1½ to 2 inches
   c. compression/ventilation ratio: 5 to 1

2. **On a child**
   a. compression rate: 80 per minute
   b. depth of compression: approximately 1 to 1½ inches
   c. compression/ventilation ratio: 5 to 1

Review Questions

Select the correct answer for each of the following questions. There is only *one* correct answer for each.

1. An infant's heartbeat should be palpated:
    a. at the carotid arteries.
    b. at the radial arteries.
    c. at the femoral arteries.
    d. at the brachial arteries.

2. In performing CPR, the chest of the infant should be compressed:
    a. ½ to ¾ inches.
    b. ½ to 1 inch.
    c. 1½ to 2 inches.
    d. 2 to 2½ inches.

3. When performing CPR on an infant, the rate of compression should be:
    a. 12 per minute.
    b. 60 per minute.
    c. 60 to 80 per minute.
    d. 80 to 100 per minute.

4. How many times should the EMT inflate the lungs of an infant before starting CPR?
    a. 1.
    b. 2.
    c. 3.
    d. 4.

5. While performing 2-operator CPR, when should the ventilator deliver the major portion of the breath?
    a. During the fifth downstroke.
    b. During the fourth upstroke.
    c. Between the fifth and first strokes.
    d. Whenever possible.

6. Which is the correct ratio for CPR with 2 persons?
    a. 1 ventilation per 5 compressions.
    b. 1 ventilation per 15 compressions.
    c. 2 ventilations per 5 compressions.
    d. 2 ventilations per 15 compressions.

7. When giving 1-operator CPR to an adult, the operator should give the chest compressions at a rate of:
    a. 12 per minute.
    b. 15 per minute.
    c. 60 per minute.
    d. 80 per minute.

8. When giving 1-operator CPR to an adult, the operator alternates between compressions and ventilations in a ratio of:
   a. 10 compressions, then 2 ventilations.
   b. 20 compressions, then 1 ventilation.
   c. 60 compressions, then 2 ventilations.
   d. 15 compressions, then 2 ventilations.

9. If a lone rescuer finds a non-breathing and pulseless victim lying face down at the scene of an auto accident, and the rescuer suspects that the victim has a back injury, which of the following should the rescuer do?
   a. Turn the victim as a unit and begin CPR.
   b. Turn the victim's head to one side and begin CPR.
   c. Do nothing and wait until help arrives.
   d. Attempt to apply CPR with the victim in the face-down position.

10. If cardiac arrest occurs due to a crushing injury to the chest:
    a. you should only give pulmonary resuscitation.
    b. give CPR but don't use as much pressure.
    c. do not give CPR for any reason.
    d. give CPR understanding that this could compound the injuries.

11. Artificial circulation is produced by compressing the chest, which squeezes the heart between:
    a. the clavicle and the scapula.
    b. the sternum and the spine.
    c. the clavicle and the spine.
    d. the sternum and the xiphoid process.

12. Complications which may result from cardiac compressions, even when performed properly, include:
    a. punctured lungs.
    b. fracture of the sternum.
    c. fractured ribs and sternum.
    d. all of the above.

13. The pulse of an arrest victim should be checked:
    a. immediately after opening the airway.
    b. after the first 4 ventilations.
    c. after the first 2 ventilations.
    d. before you start ventilations.

14. While performing chest compressions on an adult victim, the operator's hands should be:
    a. on the upper third of the sternum.
    b. 2 to 3 fingers above the lower tip of the sternum.
    c. on the middle third of the sternum.
    d. at any area of the sternum, without touching the ribs.

15. Of the following, the best procedure to follow when vomiting occurs during resuscitation, and suction equipment is not available, is to:
    a. insert a naso-gastric tube.
    b. pause for a moment until the patient appears quiet again, then resume mouth-to-mouth ventilation.
    c. switch to mouth-to-nose ventilation.
    d. turn the patient's head to the side, sweep out the mouth, and resume CPR.

16. Clinical death occurs:
    a. at the moment spontaneous circulation ceases.
    b. at the moment spontaneous ventilation ceases.
    c. at the moment both spontaneous ventilation and circulation cease.
    d. 4 to 6 minutes after all signs of life disappear.

17. Due to the size of an infant and the development of his internal organs, when performing CPR, chest compressions should be given:
    a. at the mid-sternum.
    b. to the left of the sternum.
    c. at the lower one third of the sternum.
    d. none of these.

18. Between clinical death and the onset of biological death:
    a. only seconds exist.
    b. 1 to 2 minutes exist.
    c. 4 to 6 minutes exist.
    d. 10 minutes exist.

19. Which of the following groups of symptoms are indicators of cardiac arrest?
    a. No respiration, weak carotid pulse, pupils reacting to light.
    b. No respiration, weak carotid pulse, dilated pupils.
    c. No respiration, no carotid pulse, dilated pupils.
    d. Shallow respiration, no carotid pulse, constricted pupils.

20. When performing CPR on an infant, chest compressions should be given with:
    a. both hands.
    b. the heel of 1 hand.
    c. the tips of 2 fingers.
    d. the fist of 1 hand.

21. CPR can be performed on an infant:
    a. by 1 operator.
    b. while holding the infant.
    c. while the operator is walking or sitting.
    d. all of the above.

22. The primary purpose of CPR is to:
    a. prevent biological death.
    b. prevent clinical death.
    c. restore spontaneous circulation.
    d. restore spontaneous respiration.

23. Which of the following conditions must exist before you attempt to perform CPR?
    a. Permanent brain damage has occurred.
    b. Ventilation and carotid pulses are absent.
    c. The victim's pupils are dilated.
    d. The victim has shallow respirations.

24. Under which of the following conditions is external cardiac compression too hazardous to perform?
    a. If the patient has numerous rib fractures and a "flail" chest.
    b. If a neck injury is present.
    c. Following open heart surgery.
    d. None of the above.

25. What should you do if you hear or feel rib fractures while administering cardiac compressions?
    a. Stop compressions, as the lung may become punctured.
    b. Move your hands higher on the sternum.
    c. Reduce the amount of force you are using.
    d. Don't stop. Once started, CPR should not be discontinued.

26. To determine cardiac arrest, you should check for spontaneous circulation by feeling for the:
    a. carotid or radial pulses.
    b. radial or femoral pulses.
    c. radial or temporal pulses.
    d. carotid or femoral pulses.

27. CPR can be discontinued under which of these circumstances?
    a. When the operator thinks the patient will not survive.
    b. When the operator suspects that the victim may suffer permanent brain damage.
    c. When the operator is exhausted and physically unable to continue.
    d. When an ambulance attendant states that the victim is dead.

28. A patient has been in cardiac arrest for 2 minutes and his pupils are dilated. You should:
    a. assume the patient is dead.
    b. perform CPR.
    c. transport the patient rapidly to the hospital if it is no more than 5 minutes away.
    d. suspect a head injury also.

29. When placing your hands on an adult patient's sternum to perform cardiac compressions, you should:
    a. hold the fingers of your bottom hand in a fist formation with top hand fingers curved upward.
    b. allow your fingers to conform to the patient's chest.
    c. place your hands in whatever position is comfortable.
    d. hold your fingers outward and as high as possible.

30. CPR should be continued until:
    a. additional help arrives.
    b. you think the patient is really dead.
    c. biological death occurs.
    d. the victim is pronounced dead by a physician.

31. You respond to a call and determine that a victim is in cardiac arrest. The spectators indicate that between 10 and 20 minutes have elapsed since he first "got sick." You should:
    a. start CPR immediately.
    b. not start CPR, but call for the police and for the medical examiner.
    c. start CPR on a perfunctory basis so relatives see effort, move the patient to the ambulance, then discontinue.
    d. wait until additional help arrives before starting CPR.

32. If a patient complains when you start CPR on him:
    a. he doesn't know what he's doing, so continue in the proper manner.
    b. push harder—he'll stop in a while.
    c. insert an oropharyngeal airway.
    d. you shouldn't be giving this patient CPR.

33. Except under special circumstances, once CPR is started it should not be discontinued for more than:
    a. 5 seconds.
    b. 10 seconds.
    c. 20 seconds.
    d. 30 seconds.

34. Properly performed, CPR can be effectively given to a patient:
    a. sitting in a dental chair.
    b. sitting trapped in a vehicle.
    c. only in a horizontal position.
    d. all of the above.

35. Which of the following ratios of compressions to ventilations should a single rescuer use when performing CPR on an infant?
    a. 1 to 5.
    b. 5 to 1.
    c. 15 to 2.
    d. 15 to 4.

36. When performing CPR on an infant, you should use:
    a. less pressure and a faster compression rate than for an adult.
    b. less pressure and a slower compression rate than for an adult.
    c. the same pressure and compression rate as for an adult.
    d. less pressure and the same compression rate as for an adult.

37. When cardiac arrest has occurred, and you are alone, you must remember to ventilate the patient:
    a. with greater air pressure than if there were no cardiac arrest.
    b. before starting the cardiac compressions.
    c. 4 times for every 5 cardiac compressions.
    d. as soon as you have started cardiac compressions.

38. Keeping the heel of the hand lightly in contact with the chest during the relaxation phase of cardiac compression is important because:
    a. over-expansion of the chest is avoided.
    b. correct hand position can be maintained.
    c. stomach distention can be prevented.
    d. the heartbeat can be felt.

39. You enter a house where you find a victim in respiratory and circulatory arrest. He is in bed. You should:
    a. immediately start CPR in the bed.
    b. go for a backboard, slip it under the victim, and start CPR.
    c. move the victim to the floor and start CPR.
    d. pronounce the victim dead and call the medical examiner.

40. "Closed cardiac" or "external cardiac" compression is performed:
    a. in place of mouth-to-mouth resuscitation.
    b. in place of a pressure-cycled resuscitator.
    c. to provide artificial circulation of the blood.
    d. to stimulate the electrical impulses of the heart.

41. In providing CPR for an adult, the EMT should compress the sternum about:
    a. 4 inches.
    b. 3 to 4 inches.
    c. 1½ to 2 inches.
    d. 1 inch.

42. In providing artificial circulation to an adult, when 2 EMTs are working, the sternum is compressed:
    a. at the rate of about 30 per minute.
    b. at the rate of about 60 per minute.
    c. at the rate of about 80 per minute.
    d. at whatever rate is comfortable.

Answers to Review Questions

1: d. The heartbeat of an infant should be palpated at the brachial arteries.

2: b. An infant's chest should be compressed between ½ and 1 inch.

3: d. The rate of compression with an infant should be between 80 and 100 per minute.

4: d. After determining that an infant is unresponsive, that the airway is open, and that there is no air exchange, the EMT should provide 4 puffs of air from his cheeks.

5: c. A double-sized breath should be interposed between the fifth and first strokes.

6: a. The correct ratio of ventilations to compressions with 2 operators is 1 ventilation per 5 compressions.

7: d. When 1 operator performs CPR, compressions should be performed at the rate of 80 per minute.

8: d. The ratio of compressions to ventilations when 1 operator is performing CPR is 15 compressions to 2 ventilations.

9: a. Because respiration and circulation are the EMT's first priority, the victim should be turned as a unit and CPR begun.

10: d. CPR should be started, if physically possible, regardless of the patient's injuries—the EMT has no other choice.

11: b. Artificial circulation results when the heart is squeezed between the patient's sternum and spine.

12: d. All of these injuries can be caused by properly performed chest compressions.

13: b. The carotid artery should be palpated to determine if spontaneous circulation is present after the patient has been hyperventilated with 4 double-sized breaths.

14: b. The hands of the EMT performing chest compressions should be 2 to 3 fingers above the lower tip of the sternum so no pressure is placed on the xiphoid process.

15: d. Should vomiting occur, you should turn the patient's head to one side, sweep out the vomitus with your fingers, and continue CPR as indicated.

16: c. Clinical death occurs when both spontaneous ventilation and circulation cease.

17: a. An infant's chest should be compressed at mid-sternum.

18: c. Biological death of the brain and nerve cells will begin 4 to 6 minutes after clinical death.

19: c. No respiration, no carotid pulse, and dilated pupils are indicators of cardiac arrest.

20: c. The tips of 2 fingers should be used to compress the sternum of an infant.

21: d. CPR can be given to an infant under all of these conditions.

22: a. The primary purpose of CPR is to prevent biological death by providing artificial circulation and ventilation.

23: b. CPR should not be performed unless there is no respiration and both carotid pulses are absent.

24: d. CPR should be performed regardless of the patient's injuries or condition.

25: d. CPR must be continued in the normal manner, as it takes priority over any other treatment.

26: d. Palpate the carotid or femoral pulses to determine if a patient is in cardiac arrest. These are major arteries, and are easily palpated.

27: c. CPR can be discontinued only if the operator is exhausted and is physically unable to continue.

28: b. You should begin CPR immediately.

29: d. You should hold your fingers outward and as high as possible so they do not touch the patient's chest. Compressions should be performed with the heel of the hand.

30: d. CPR should be continued until the patient is pronounced dead by a physician.

31: a. Start CPR immediately after determining that both spontaneous respiration and circulation are absent.

32: d. CPR should not be performed unless both spontaneous respiration and circulation are absent.

33: a. CPR should not be discontinued for more than 5 seconds, except under certain extraordinary circumstances. When compressions are discontinued, blood flow stops.

34: c. CPR can only be performed when the patient is horizontal (supine) on a firm, unyielding surface so that the heart can be squeezed between the sternum and spine.

35: b. The proper ratio of compressions to ventilations when CPR is performed on an infant is the same as that when 2 operators treat an adult—5 compressions for each ventilation—but at a faster rate.

36: a. Chest compressions are performed on an infant with less pressure and at a faster rate than for an adult.

37: b. You should hyperventilate the patient with 4 double-sized breaths before starting artificial circulation.

38: b. The operator performing chest compressions can maintain the proper position of his hands by keeping them lightly in contact with the patient's chest at all times.

39: c. Quickly moving the patient to the floor will save valuable time. A backboard can be brought from the ambulance and placed under the patient while CPR is in progress.

40: c. Chest compressions are performed to manually or artificially circulate the patient's blood.

41: c. You should compress the sternum of an adult 1½ to 2 inches.

42: b. When 2 operators perform CPR, the chest is compressed 60 times per minute.

Practical Applications

Assume you are part of a 2-person ambulance crew. Describe what action you would take, and why, in the following situations.

1. A child has put a hairpin into an electric wall socket. When you arrive he is unconscious and not breathing, but is still clinging to the hairpin in the socket.

2. A young swimmer has been pulled from the bottom of a pool. He is not breathing and has no pulse.

3. You and a friend, who is also an EMT, are shopping when an elderly woman collapses nearby. You both rush to her aid. She is not breathing and has no pulse at either carotid artery. You send someone to call for an ambulance.

4. A frantic young mother calls to report that her newborn has stopped breathing. Upon arrival at the scene you find the mother has begun mouth-to-mouth resuscitation. You immediately check for a pulse and none can be felt.

5. A car has hit a pole. Witnesses tell you that the accident just happened. Your primary survey of the driver indicates widely dilated pupils, the absence of both carotid pulses, and no ventilations. The patient is being held upright by the steering wheel, and a rescue company is on the way.

6. You start CPR on a man that has been hit by a car. As you compress his sternum, blood flows from his thigh.

7. You enter a bedroom to find a police officer performing 1-operator CPR on an elderly man. The patient's wife tells you that he has been very sick and asks, "Why can't you let him die with dignity?"

8. A middle-aged woman has collapsed in a movie theater. There are no ventilations, both carotid pulses are absent, her eyes are widely dilated and do not respond to light. She is wearing a medi-alert necklace stating she is a diabetic.

9. As you provide the 4 stepped ventilations to a man with no pulse or ventilations, your partner tells you that the victim's chest will not rise. You encounter no resistance to your ventilations.

10. You find a patient with a weak, rapid pulse, who is not breathing.

11. You arrive at a home and find a 4-year-old male child cyanotic and "crowing."

Chapter 8

WOUNDS, CONTROL OF BLEEDING, AND SHOCK

Comprehensive Questions

1. What are the 4 types of open wounds? Describe each one.

2. What are the techniques available to the EMT for the control of bleeding? In what order should they be used?

3. How does direct pressure serve to control bleeding?

4. Under what conditions should pressure points be used in the control of bleeding?

5. What are the rules for the use of a tourniquet? Explain the reasons for each.

6. Why should an impaled object not be removed?

7. What is shock? Why is it a life-threatening condition?

8. What are the stages of shock and the signs that accompany each?

9. Why is it inappropriate to rely on blood pressure alone as a means of determining that a patient is in shock?

10. Why is treatment for shock indicated in any sudden medical emergency or trauma regardless of whether a clear clinical picture is present?

Performance Skills

1. Control severe hemorrhage with the application of direct pressure.

2. Control severe hemorrhage by exerting pressure at the proper pressure point.

3. Control severe hemorrhage with the use of a tourniquet.

4. Treat a patient for epistaxis (nosebleed).

5. Control bleeding from, and properly dress and bandage, an impaled object.

6. Properly dress and bandage an evisceration.

7. Control bleeding from, and properly dress and bandage, an amputation. Prepare the amputated part for transport.

8. Assess the presence of shock and carry out proper treatment.

Reference Data

1. **Types of wounds**
   a. contusion
   b. abrasion
   c. laceration
   d. avulsion
   e. puncture

2. **Steps to control bleeding**
   a. direct pressure and elevation
   b. pressure point
   c. tourniquet

3. **Shock** results from decreased cardiac output caused by:
   a. loss of fluid volume
   b. damage to the heart
   c. dilation of the circulatory system

4. **Types of shock**
   a. hemorrhagic: blood loss
   b. respiratory: inadequate oxygen supply
   c. neurogenic: nervous system failure or intense pain
   d. psychogenic: emotional stress
   e. cardiogenic: inadequate functioning of the heart
   f. septic: severe infection
   g. metabolic: dehydration or changes in blood chemistry
   h. anaphylactic: allergic reaction

5. **Stages of shock and accompanying clinical picture**
   a. early (compensated): Skin is pale and moist; patient is weak and anxious; pulse rate is elevated; respiration rate is elevated.
   b. late (progressive): Increased tachycardia and weakness; blood pressure falls rapidly; body temperature decreases; patient is unconscious; respirations are shallow; patient is cyanotic.

Review Questions

Select the correct answer for each of the following questions. There is only *one* correct answer for each.

1. Internal bleeding should be suspected when a patient:
    a. exhibits the signs of shock with no external hemorrhage.
    b. is vomiting blood that has the appearance of "coffee grounds."
    c. has a stiff, board-like abdomen.
    d. All of the above.

2. A person in shock, but still conscious, should be given:
    a. clear liquids.
    b. coffee or tea.
    c. fluids with special electrolytes.
    d. nothing by mouth.

3. An avulsion is a wound where:
    a. there is snagging and tearing of tissue.
    b. the skin and underlying tissue are disrupted by a sharp pointed object.
    c. a flap of skin and tissue is hanging or torn loose.
    d. the skin surface is abraded with penetration of all layers of the skin.

4. An incision is a wound:
    a. usually made by a sharp-edged object.
    b. resulting from snagging and tearing of tissue.
    c. with rough, ragged edges of skin and underlying tissue.
    d. where large flaps of skin and tissue are torn loose.

5. Which of the following is an open wound?
    a. Avulsion.
    b. Puncture.
    c. Laceration.
    d. All of the above.

6. An amputated part should be:
    a. carefully replaced on its original site, dressed, and bandaged firmly.
    b. carefully replaced on its original site, and secured with moist dressings and bandages.
    c. rinsed off, kept cold, and transported with the patient, if possible.
    d. placed in a sterile saline solution and transported with the patient.

7. If there is a sizable foreign body protruding from a wound you should:
   a. remove it, to prevent infection.
   b. remove it, to prevent it going deeper.
   c. remove it, otherwise a pressure dressing cannot be applied.
   d. leave it, because removal may cause serious bleeding.

8. Arterial bleeding should be suspected when:
   a. the blood is bright red and is flowing steadily from the wound.
   b. the blood is bright red and is spurting from the wound.
   c. the blood is dark maroon and is flowing steadily from the wound.
   d. the blood is dark maroon and is spurting from the wound.

9. The procedure of choice to control bleeding from an extremity is:
   a. tourniquet and elevation.
   b. direct pressure and elevation.
   c. pressure points.
   d. bandaging.

10. When treating a nosebleed, you should keep the patient in a sitting position, keep the patient quiet, and:
    a. apply pressure by squeezing the nostrils.
    b. place a bandage between the upper lip and gum and have the patient draw his upper lip taut to produce pressure.
    c. apply ice wrapped in a cloth to the nose.
    d. all of the above.

11. Which of the following is a possible indication of internal bleeding?
    a. Reduced pulse rate and soft stomach/abdomen.
    b. Increased pulse rate and rigid stomach/abdomen.
    c. Reduced pulse rate and dilated pupils.
    d. Increased pulse rate and soft stomach/abdomen.

12. If a tourniquet must be used, you should:
    a. tighten it slowly, until the bleeding stops.
    b. never cover it.
    c. mark "TK" on forehead or tag so that other medical personnel know it is there.
    d. all of the above.

13. Which of the following groups of signs and symptoms indicates that a patient may be in shock?
    a. Slow, strong pulse; dizziness; cold perspiration; nausea.
    b. Rapid, weak pulse; cold, clammy skin; pallor; shallow breathing.
    c. Blank expression; cold extremities; regular breathing.
    d. Blank expression; chills; unconsciousness; dry skin.

14. Which of the following is not an emergency care procedure for the treatment of a person in shock?
    a. Keep the patient lying down with the legs elevated.
    b. Give the patient water to drink.
    c. Prevent the loss of body heat by putting blankets under and over the patient.
    d. Administer oxygen.

15. You have arrived at the scene of an automobile accident. One of the victims has an open gash on his forehead which is bleeding. What should you do?
    a. Apply a sterile dressing with a loose bandage.
    b. Apply pressure to the carotid artery.
    c. Apply pressure to the subclavian artery.
    d. Apply a sterile dressing with a snug bandage.

16. A young male has been cut above the ankle by a lawn mower blade. If hemorrhage cannot be controlled by direct pressure, you should apply pressure on:
    a. the dorsalis pedis artery.
    b. the subclavian artery.
    c. the temporal artery.
    d. the femoral artery.

17. An EMT finds an accident victim with an amputated leg. If other means of controlling hemorrhage fail, the recommended treatment is:
    a. to apply a tourniquet about 2 inches above the stump.
    b. apply a sterile dressing and a snug bandage over the stump.
    c. transport immediately.
    d. irrigate the stump with sterile water.

18. In cases of severe blood loss you should administer:
    a. 25 percent oxygen.
    b. 50 percent oxygen.
    c. 100 percent oxygen.
    d. no oxygen; the need is for blood.

19. After the sudden onset of a medical emergency, or severe trauma, you should treat for shock:
    a. when a pattern of signs and symptoms develops.
    b. only in severe cases displaying all signs and symptoms.
    c. routinely—not waiting for signs or symptoms to develop.
    d. only after treating all other problems.

20. A person in shock will exhibit the following signs:
    a. decreasing pulse rate, and decreasing BP.
    b. increasing pulse rate, and increasing BP.
    c. increasing pulse rate, and decreasing BP.
    d. decreasing pulse rate, and increasing BP.

21. Psychogenic shock is a reaction of the nervous sytem to certain stimuli such as the sight of blood. This type of shock:
    a. is a true emergency, requiring medical attention.
    b. may be reversed by administering oxygen.
    c. is not a true emergency, but must be treated promptly.
    d. is self-correcting unless other problems are present.

22. An anaphylactic reaction may, within seconds, cause all of the following *except:*
    a. constricted pupils.
    b. weak, imperceptible pulse.
    c. difficulty breathing.
    d. itching of skin, with or without hives.

23. Of the following, the only really effective treatment an EMT is authorized to provide for a patient in anaphylactic shock is:
    a. an injection of epinephrine.
    b. administration of 100 percent oxygen.
    c. placing the patient in the Trendelenberg position.

24. In treating a conscious patient suffering from cardiogenic shock, you should:
    a. transport in a semi-sitting position.
    b. transport in the Trendelenberg position.
    c. transport in a prone position.
    d. transport in the coma position.

25. In certain rare situations you might elect to use a tourniquet without attempting other methods of hemorrhage control. Such a situation would be:
    a. if there is uncontrollable hemorrhage from an amputated limb.
    b. if there are multiple wounds which are hemorrhaging severely.
    c. if there are several patients in need of treatment, one of whom is hemorrhaging severely.
    d. any of the above.

26. Use of a tourniquet to stop bleeding of an extremity is a last resort because a tourniquet:
    a. is painful.
    b. doesn't always work.
    c. may cause loss of the limb.

27. Although any place where a blood vessel can be pressed against a bony surface is a pressure point, the 2 most commonly used are located:
    a. at the medial upper arm and the medial thigh.
    b. at the medial upper arm and the groin.
    c. at the neck and the groin.
    d. at the posterior upper arm and the medial thigh.

28. An open wound characterized by capillary bleeding is called:
    a. abrasion.
    b. an avulsion.
    c. a contusion.
    d. a laceration.

29. A collection of blood in the tissues resulting from injury or a broken blood vessel is called:
    a. an avulsion.
    b. a hematoma.
    c. an incision.
    d. an abrasion.

30. When treating severe, closed, soft tissue injuries, swelling and bleeding below the skin can be controlled by:
    a. applying warmth, and a snug bandage for mild pressure.
    b. applying cold, and transporting immediately.
    c. applying cold, and a snug bandage for mild pressure.
    d. applying direct pressure and elevating.

31. Which of the following describes bleeding from a vein?
    a. Bright red, flowing steadily.
    b. Bright red, spurting.
    c. Dark maroon, flowing steadily.
    d. Dark maroon, spurting.

32. An impaled foreign object in a wound:
    a. should be carefully removed by the EMT to allow control of bleeding and proper bandaging.
    b. eliminates the possibility of the EMT using direct pressure.
    c. should be left in place and stabilized.
    d. should never be cut down or shortened.

33. Which of the following types of shock is most likely to cause swelling of the face, tongue, and respiratory tract?
    a. Septic.
    b. Metabolic.
    c. Anaphylactic.
    d. Hypovolemic.

34. Administering oxygen in the ambulance is essential:
    a. only if the patient has an open wound.
    b. only if the patient has a closed wound.
    c. whether the wound is open or closed.

35. A small patient has a BP of 90/60, and a full pulse of 86. His condition is possibly:
    a. a normal state of health.
    b. hypovolemic shock.
    c. anaphylactic shock.
    d. metabolic shock.

36. Which of these materials should *never* be used for a tourniquet?
    a. Piece of rope.
    b. Folded handkerchief.
    c. Triangular bandage.
    d. Belt.

37. Which of the following is a closed wound?
    a. Puncture.
    b. Avulsion.
    c. Laceration.
    d. Contusion.

38. Which of the following is most susceptible to tetanus?
    a. Laceration.
    b. Amputation.
    c. Incision.
    d. Puncture.

39. Formation of an air embolism is most commonly seen in:
    a. laceration of the carotid artery.
    b. laceration of the jugular vein.
    c. a soft tissue injury.
    d. a femoral fracture.

40. Which of the following is an open wound?
    a. Contusion.
    b. Hematoma.
    c. Laceration.

41. Which of the following is the name for an open wound that has jagged skin edges and is bleeding freely?
    a. Laceration.
    b. Abrasion.
    c. Incision.
    d. Puncture.

42. Which artery is the *least* dependable for taking a pulse in a patient who appears to be in shock?
    a. Carotid.
    b. Femoral.
    c. Radial.
    d. Brachial.

43. Which of the following is the most dependable location for taking a pulse?
    a. Radial artery.
    b. Brachial artery.
    c. Carotid artery.
    d. Dorsalis pedis artery.

44. After controlling the bleeding from a serious open wound of the leg, you should:
    a. immobilize and keep the injured part on the same level as the rest of the body.
    b. immobilize and lower the injured part.
    c. immobilize and elevate the injured part.
    d. keep the injured part on the same level as the rest of the body.

45. In a case of severe hemorrhage, if no dressing is handy, you should:
    a. use a pressure point.
    b. quickly go and find one, or a substitute such as a sanitary napkin or clean cloth.
    c. use your bare hand.
    d. use your bare hand after washing with soap.

46. Control of severe hemorrhage is:
    a. only attempted after a full survey of the patient.
    b. only critical if low pulse and blood pressure are found.
    c. a high priority of treatment.
    d. all of the above.

47. The soft tissue injury caused by the impact of a blunt object is called:
    a. a contusion.
    b. a concussion.
    c. an abrasion.
    d. an avulsion.

48. Which of the following types of shock results from a failure of the nervous system?
    a. Hemorrhagic.
    b. Neurogenic.
    c. Psychogenic.
    d. Anaphylactic.

49. If a tourniquet must be used, it must be:
    a. put on tightly and left on, only to be removed by a physician.
    b. put on, tightened for 20 minutes, released for 10, etc.
    c. put on and tightened for 15 minutes and released for 5, etc.
    d. taken off after 1 hour.

50. Which of the following types of shock results from an inadequate oxygen supply?
    a. Hemorrhagic.
    b. Respiratory.
    c. Metabolic.
    d. Neurogenic.

51. When giving emergency care to patients in shock, it is important to maintain an adequate oxygen supply to the brain. To help in doing this, you can:
    a. elevate the lower extremities.
    b. slightly elevate the upper part of the body.
    c. tilt the entire body up at the head.
    d. elevate the lower extremities and trunk of the body.

52. Which type of shock can result from the loss of 2 pints of blood in an average-sized adult male?
    a. Septic shock.
    b. Metabolic shock.
    c. Cardiogenic shock.
    d. Hemorrhagic shock.

53. When treating patients in shock:
    a. oxygen should always be given.
    b. oxygen is not an indicated treatment.
    c. oxygen is only an indicated treatment if respiratory difficulty or arrest occur.
    d. oxygen is only of peripheral benefit and should only be administered after all other treatment.

54. In emergency medicine, shock means:
    a. sudden hemorrhage.
    b. a CVA.
    c. a stroke.
    d. collapse of the cardiovascular system.

55. Anaphylactic shock can be caused by:
    a. insect stings or bites.
    b. ingesting foods or drugs.
    c. injecting drugs.
    d. all of these.

Answers to Review Questions

1: d. All of these are indicators of internal bleeding.

2: d. You should give a patient in shock nothing by mouth.

3: c. An avulsion occurs when a flap of skin or tissue is hanging loose or torn off.

4: a. An incision is a wound made by a sharp-edged object.

5: d. Avulsions, punctures, and lacerations are all open wounds.

6: c. An amputated part should be rinsed off, kept cold, and transported with the patient, if possible.

7: d. An impaled object should not be removed. Removal could cause further tissue damage and increased hemorrhage.

8: b. Arterial bleeding is indicated by bright red blood that spurts with each contraction of the heart.

9: b. The best method to control bleeding from an extremity, and the least damaging, is the use of direct pressure and elevation.

10: a. Apply pressure by squeezing the nostrils.

11: b. An increased pulse rate and a rigid stomach or abdomen are indicators of possible internal bleeding.

12: d. All of these are proper techniques when using a tourniquet.

13: b. The indicators of shock include a rapid but weak pulse; cold, clammy skin; pallor; and shallow, often irregular respiration.

14: b. The EMT should not usually administer anything by mouth.

15: d. Bleeding from a head wound should be treated with a sterile dressing bandage snug enough to control the bleeding.

16: d. Since the bleeding is above the ankle, you should use the femoral pressure point.

17: a Apply a tourniquet about 2 inches above the stump.

18: c. You should administer 100 percent oxygen to compensate for the loss of oxygen-carrying red blood cells.

19: c. You should treat for shock routinely to prevent the onset of shock, which can be life-threatening.

20: c. A patient in shock will have increased pulse rate with a decreasing blood pressure.

21: d. Psychogenic shock is usually self-correcting as the body adjusts to the sudden dilation of the blood vessels.

22: a. Constricted pupils are *not* a result of anaphylactic shock.

23: b. Since anaphylaxis can be combatted only by drug therapy, an EMT can only treat this condition with 100 percent oxygen.

24: a. A conscious victim of cardiogenic shock should be transported in a semi-sitting position with the administration of oxygen.

25: d. All of these situations present conditions under which you may decide to apply a tourniquet first.

26: c. A tourniquet, if left on for an extended period, can cause the loss of the portion of the limb distal to it.

27: b. The 2 most effective pressure points are the brachial and femoral, located inside the upper arm and at the groin.

28: a. An abrasion or "scrape" usually covers a larger area than other kinds of wounds, and is characterized by capillary bleeding.

29: b. A hematoma is a pool of blood caused when vessels are disrupted without the continuity of the skin being disturbed.

30: c. The EMT should apply cold to reduce swelling and apply a snug bandage. An extremity should also be immobilized.

31: c. Venous bleeding is usually dark in color with a steady flow.

32: c. An impaled object should *not* be removed. It should be left in place and stabilized to avoid further injury.

33: c. These signs are indicators of anaphylactic shock.

34: c. Oxygen should be administered to prevent shock regardless of the type of wound.

35: a. This patient is probably in a normal healthy state. A strong, full pulse of 86 indicates good health, and many small people have a normal blood pressure below 100.

36: a. Rope, wire, or other narrow substances should *not* be used as tourniquets since they can cause nerve and vessel damage.

37: d. A contusion is a bruise. Bleeding is contained below the skin, so it is a closed wound.

38: d. Puncture wounds are most susceptible to tetanus due to their depth and usual lack of bleeding.

39: b. Air embolism can result from lacerations of the jugular vein.

40: c. A laceration is an open wound.

41: a. A laceration has jagged edges while an incision has straight clean edges. Both can bleed freely.

42: c. The radial artery, while most commonly used, is the least reliable since it is most distal from the heart and is small in diameter.

43: c. The carotid pulse is the most reliable.

44: c. You should immobilize the extremity and elevate it.

45: c. Use your bare hand—do not waste valuable time washing or looking for a dressing of any kind.

46: c. Control of hemorrhage is always given one of the highest priorities of treatment.

47: a. A contusion is a soft tissue injury caused by a blunt object.

48: b. Neurogenic shock is the type that is caused by a failure of the nervous system.

49: a. If a tourniquet must be used, it must be put on tightly, left on, and only be removed by a physician.

50: b. Respiratory shock is caused by an inadequate oxygen supply.

51: a. Elevation of the lower extremities increases the amount of blood available to the vital organs of the chest and head.

52: d. Hemorrhagic shock results from excessive blood loss.

53: a. Oxygen should be given to all patients in shock.

54: d. Shock is defined as a collapse of the cardiovascular system resulting in inadequate tissue perfusion.

55: d. All of these can cause the allergic reaction which produces anaphylactic shock.

Practical Applications

Consider how you would act, and why, in the following situations.

1. You are called to treat a child who has had a bicycle accident. When you arrive, the child is some 25 feet away from the accident site, sitting on a porch. He tells you he skidded on sand and fell off the bike. He remembers everything that happened. The only thing that hurts is his knee which is scraped and bleeding.

2. A young boy has run through a glass door and has suffered severe laceration of the scalp and right arm. You find him writhing in pain in a large pool of blood. You see no shards of glass in any of the wounds. Pulse is 100 and weak; respirations, 24; blood pressure is 90/40.

3. You respond to an industrial accident where a worker's forearm has been amputated above the wrist by a machine. When you arrive, the stump is still bleeding heavily. Vitals are: pulse, 100 and weak; respirations, 24 and shallow; blood pressure, 80/40.

4. A young man was assaulted by a gang of youths with bats and sticks. He complained to bystanders of abdominal pain before you arrived. When you arrive, the victim is semi-conscious and pale. Pulse is 110 and thready; respirations are 24; blood pressure is 92/62.

5. In a motor vehicle accident the passenger was thrown from the car that hit the guard rail. The head has a closed, depressed fracture. Blood pressure is 160/110; pulse is 50; respirations are 24.

6. You respond to an auto accident and find a young woman with a deep laceration to her right thigh. She has no other injuries. The bleeding is severe, but is not spurting. Her vitals are: pulse, 90; respirations, 18; blood pressure, 100/70.

7. You respond to a home accident to find a man who injured his hand while trying to unclog his lawn mower. His right index finger has been amputated at the first joint. The bleeding has been stopped by a towel wrapped tightly around the finger. The avulsed finger tip is found nearby. His pulse is 80; respirations are 20; blood pressure is 110/70. His skin is pale.

8. A 45-year-old woman has been injured in a factory. Portions of the intestines are protruding from the abdominal cavity. Blood pressure is 90/60; pulse is 120; respirations are 24.

9. A piece of metal, which has penetrated the cheek of a 25-year-old male, is still embedded. Control of bleeding by usual methods is not possible. Blood pressure is 130/80; pulse is 110; respirations are 18.

Chapter 9

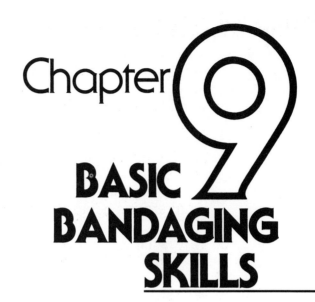

BASIC BANDAGING SKILLS

Comprehensive Questions

1. What are the differences between a dressing and a bandage?

2. What are the purposes of dressing and bandaging a wound?

3. What are the materials available to the EMT for dressing and bandaging a wound? What are the advantages and disadvantages of each?

4. What are the basic elements of a good bandage?

5. Why is it important to check the patient's skin color and temperature distal to the bandage periodically?

6. Why should a dressing rarely be removed from a wound once it has been applied?

Performance Skills

1. Select the appropriate dressing for any wound.

2. Apply dressings and an appropriate bandage to each of the following bleeding injuries:
   a. the arm or leg.
   b. the elbow or knee.
   c. the hand or foot.
   d. the fingers or toes.
   e. the shoulder or hip.
   f. the trunk of the body.
   g. the forehead and scalp.
   h. the ear and cheek.
   i. the mandible.
   j. the neck.

3. Apply a sling and swathe.

Reference Data

GENERAL RULES FOR DRESSING AND BANDAGING ANY WOUND.

1. The dressing must adequately cover the wound.

2. Apply enough bandage to adequately protect the dressing.

3. Do *not* bandage more of the body than is necessary.

4. A bandage must be firm and snug but *not* so tight as to restrict circulation.

5. A bandage should be tied or fastened so it will not move.

6. Never tie knots so that they are on the skin.

7. Avoid placing knots at the patient's back.

8. Whenever possible, avoid applying tape directly to the skin.

9. There should be no loose ends that could become caught when the patient is moved.

10. Compare the circulation, skin color, and temperature above and below the bandaged area.

11. Avoid covering fingertips and toes so that they can be periodically checked for proper circulation.

Review Questions

Select the correct answer for each of the following questions. There is only *one* correct answer for each.

1. A bandage should:
    a. just cover the dressing.
    b. extend 8 to 12 inches beyond the dressing on each side.
    c. extend sufficiently beyond the dressing to prevent dirt from reaching the wound or dressing.
    d. be loosely wound to allow air to enter.

2. If you have applied a pressure bandage and the bleeding hasn't stopped, you should:
    a. immediately use the pressure point.
    b. put pressure on the bandage with your hand or tighten it, being sure not to turn it into a constrictor or tourniquet.
    c. tighten it so it becomes a tourniquet.
    d. place another bandage 6 inches above the wound.

3. Removing a dressing that has been applied to a wound could cause:
    a. contamination of the wound.
    b. release of pressure on the wound.
    c. destruction of clots that have formed.
    d. all of the above.

4. When bandaging an extremity, you should:
    a. apply the bandage tightly over the fingers or toes.
    b. apply the bandage loosely over the fingers or toes.
    c. leave the fingers or toes exposed whenever possible.
    d. all of the above.

5. When treating an open wound you should first control hemorrhage, then apply a dressing and a bandage. The dressing:
    a. should be sterile if possible.
    b. forms a matrix to aid clotting.
    c. is placed directly on the wound and should not be moved once it is in place.
    d. all of the above.

6. Which of the following is *not* a function of a dressing?
    a. Absorption of blood.
    b. As a matrix for clotting.
    c. Protection from further contamination.
    d. Killing of bacteria already present in the wound.

7. Which of the following statements about dressings and bandages is *not* correct?
    a. Bandages are used to hold dressings in place.
    b. Dressings are used to hold bandages in place.
    c. Bandages need not be sterile.
    d. Dressings are used to prevent contamination.

8. After applying both a dressing and a bandage to a laceration below the patient's elbow, you should check:
    a. for changes in sensation distal to the dressing.
    b. for the presence of a pulse distal to the dressing.
    c. the dressing for continued bleeding.
    d. all of the above.

9. If blood soaks through a dressing you should:
    a. replace it with a new one.
    b. use your bare hand instead of a dressing.
    c. remove the dressing and compress a pressure point.
    d. place another dressing on top of the first one.

10. A bandage may be applied in generally the same way to *both* an elbow and which of the following?
    a. Hand.
    b. Knee.
    C. Foot.
    d. Shoulder.

11. A laceration can be properly bandaged with:
    a. a roller bandage.
    b. a self-adhering bandage.
    c. a cravat.
    d. any of the above.

12. An occlusive dressing is most commonly used on a:
    a. sucking chest wound.
    b. laceration.
    c. puncture wound.
    d. closed comminuted fracture.

13. After wetting a dressing with sterile saline solution, the "wound field" is:
    a. now open to contamination.
    b. still sterile.
    c. aseptic.
    d. anti-microbial.

14. Cotton as a dressing is:
    a. not recommended.
    b. used for epistaxis.
    c. used in packing ear injuries.
    d. helpful in stabilizing an avulsed eye.

15. In extreme cases, the EMT's hand may be used as a:
    a. compress.
    b. tourniquet.
    c. bandage.
    d. none of the above.

16. After it has been applied, a bandage made from roller gauze should be tied or taped so that:
    a. it does not unwind.
    b. it does not catch on anything as the patient is moved.
    c. it does not slide or move.
    d. all of the above.

Answers to Review Questions

1: c. A bandage should extend beyond the dressing to prevent dirt from reaching the wound or dressing.

2: b. If bleeding does not stop after a pressure bandage has been applied, put pressure on the bandage with your hand or tighten it, but make certain it does not impair circulation.

3: d. All of these can result if a dressing is removed.

4: c. You should leave the patient's fingers and toes exposed to determine that his circulation is not impaired.

5: d. All of these are true of a dressing.

6: d. A dressing cannot kill the bacteria already present in the wound.

7: b. The statement, "Dressings are used to hold bandages in place," is incorrect.

8: d. All of these are things you should check.

9: d. If a dressing becomes blood-soaked, place another on top of it. Do not remove the first one.

10: b. An elbow and a knee are bandaged in generally the same way.

11: d. Any of these materials can be used to bandage a laceration.

12: a. An occlusive dressing is most commonly used to seal a sucking chest wound.

13: a. The "wound field" is open to contamination once it has been wet with a saline solution.

14: a. Cotton is not recommended for use as a dressing because the fibers can become stuck to the wound.

15: a. In certain circumstances the EMT can and should use his hand directly on a wound to control bleeding.

16: d. All of these are reasons to tie or tape a bandage securely.

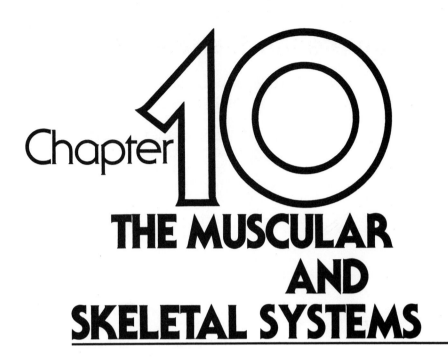

Chapter 10

THE MUSCULAR
AND
SKELETAL SYSTEMS

Comprehensive Questions

1. What are the differences between the voluntary and the involuntary muscles?

2. Explain how muscle is attached to bone and how this provides for body movement.

3. Explain the statement: "Muscles cannot push, they only pull."

4. What functions do skeletal muscles serve beyond their role in body movement?

5. List and describe the functions of the skeletal system.

6. Explain the statement: "Bones are living tissue."

7. Describe the various types of bone joints.

8. List and define the types of fractures.

9. What are the differences between fractures, sprains, strains, and dislocations?

Reference Data

1.

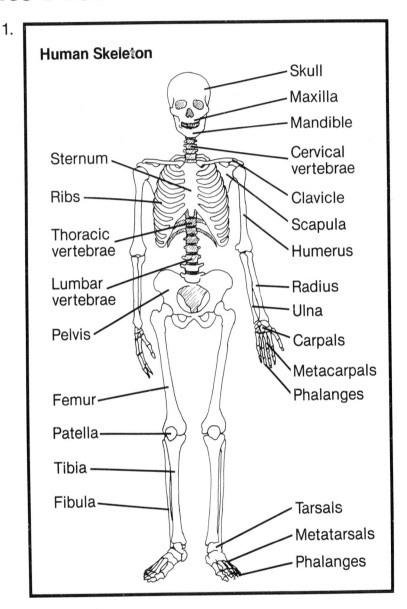

Human Skeleton

Skull

Maxilla

Mandible

Cervical vertebrae

Sternum

Clavicle

Ribs

Scapula

Thoracic vertebrae

Humerus

Lumbar vertebrae

Radius

Ulna

Pelvis

Carpals

Metacarpals

Phalanges

Femur

Patella

Tibia

Fibula

Tarsals

Metatarsals

Phalanges

2.

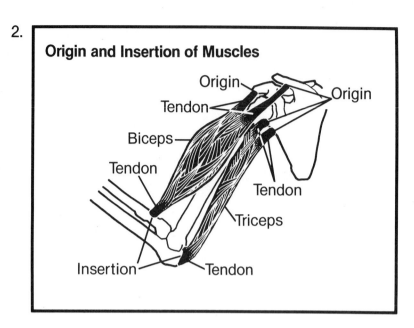

Origin and Insertion of Muscles

3. **Types of muscles**
   a. **voluntary** (striated): skeletal muscle that is under voluntary control
   b. **involuntary** (smooth): most internal organs; under control of autonomic nervous system
   c. **cardiac:** heart muscle

Review Questions

Select the correct answer for each of the following questions. There is only *one* correct answer for each.

1. Which of the following types of muscle moves bones?
    a. Smooth.
    b. Voluntary.
    c. Involuntary.

2. Skeletal muscles usually have 2 points of attachment. One is to the bone it flexes or extends. This point is called its:
    a. origin.
    b. insertion.
    c. articulation.
    d. all of these.

3. The bone of the lower leg that connects with the femur at the knee is the:
    a. radius.
    b. fibula.
    c. humerus.
    d. tibia.

4. The ribs most frequently fractured are the:
    a. second through fourth.
    b. first through fifth.
    c. fourth through tenth.
    d. eleventh and twelfth.

5. Which of the following bones connects to the humerus?
    a. Radius.
    b. Clavicle.
    c. Fibula.
    d. Tibia.

6. Located at the front of the chest is a flat bony structure that joins the ribs. This structure is called the:
    a. xiphoid process.
    b. scapula.
    c. sternum.
    d. clavicle.

7. The jaw is divided into 2 parts: the maxilla, or upper jaw, and the lower jaw, called the:
    a. clavicle.
    b. mandible.
    c. zygoma.
    d. temporal.

8. A dislocation is an injury to:
    a. a bone.
    b. a joint.
    c. a muscle.
    d. tendons.

9. Synovial fluid:
    a. protects the brain and spinal cord.
    b. lubricates the bones at a joint.
    c. is the yellowish fluid portion of the blood.
    d. may be found in the ears if the skull is fractured.

10. Involuntary muscles:
    a. contract without our conscious control.
    b. contract only when consciously controlled.
    c. are also called skeletal muscles.

11. Muscle tissue is unique because when stimulated by nerves it can:
    a. contract.
    b. expand.
    c. be sprained.
    d. be strained.

12. The biceps is an example of:
    a. smooth muscle tissue.
    b. voluntary muscle tissue.
    c. involuntary muscle tissue.
    d. cardiac muscle tissue.

13. The diaphragm is:
    a. a voluntary muscle.
    b. an involuntary muscle.
    c. both a voluntary and involuntary muscle.
    d. a cardiac muscle.

14. Which of the following muscles are voluntary?
    a. Muscles of the blood vessels.
    b. Muscles of the intestines.
    c. Muscles of the stomach.
    d. Skeletal muscles.

15. An example of a hinged joint can be found at the:
    a. sacroiliac.
    b. shoulder.
    c. knee.
    d. hip.

16. Skeletal muscles that work in opposition to others are called:
    a. collateral.
    b. compensatory.
    c. antagonistic.

17. Which one of the following is not ordinarily dislocated?
    a. Shoulder.
    b. Elbow.
    c. Clavicle.
    d. Hip.

18. An example of involuntary muscle is the:
    a. triceps.
    b. biceps.
    c. deltoid.
    d. intestinal wall.

19. Ball and socket joints allow for motion:
    a. from front to back.
    b. from side to side.
    c. in one place.
    d. in all directions.

20. The type of material which forms the end of a bone is called:
    a. periosteum.
    b. articular cartilage.
    c. compact bone.
    d. cancellous bone.

21. Generally, patients with injuries to the bones and joints require:
    a. rapid transportation to the hospital.
    b. rapid treatment for life-threatening injury.
    c. no attention until arrival at the hospital.
    d. slow, deliberate treatment and transportation.

22. The longest, heaviest bones of the human skeleton are the:
    a. femurs.
    b. ulnas.
    c. tarsals.
    d. fibulas.

23. An example of a fused joint in an adult can be found at the:
    a. cranium.
    b. shoulder.
    c. knee.

24. An example of a ball and socket joint is found at the:
    a. elbow.
    b. knee.
    c. hip.
    d. ankle.

25. Examples of "irregular bones" are:
    a. the bones of the leg.
    b. the vertebrae of the spinal column.
    c. the bones of the skull.

26. The "pelvic" bone of an adult is actually formed of how many parts of bones fused together?
    a. 1.
    b. 3.
    c. 5.
    d. 7.

27. The lower leg is made up of the:
    a. metatarsals and tarsals.
    b. tibia and metatarsals.
    c. fibula and tarsals.
    d. tibia and fibula.

28. The bones that make up the forearm are the:
    a. radius and ulna.
    b. tibia and fibula.
    c. carpals and metacarpals.
    d. scapula and humerus.

29. The rib cage is made up of:
    a. 8 pairs of ribs.
    b. 10 pairs of ribs.
    c. 12 pairs of ribs.
    d. 14 pairs of ribs.

30. The skeletal system functions to:
    a. protect vital organs.
    b. give the body support and shape.
    c. provide locomotion.
    d. all of the above.

31. The human skeleton is made up of approximately:
    a. 100 bones.
    b. 200 bones.
    c. 300 bones.
    d. 400 bones.

32. The cartilaginous structure at the inferior end of the sternum is called:
    a. the scapula.
    b. the steroid process.
    c. the xiphoid process.
    d. the clavicle.

33. Muscles can relax and contract and pull on bones, but cannot:
    a. flex a bone.
    b. extend a bone.
    c. push a bone.
    d. become wider.

34. A sprain usually occurs:
   a. at a joint.
   b. when a heavy object is lifted.
   c. when the continuity of a bone is broken.
   d. when a fracture is improperly splinted.

35. The tough, connective tissues that attach bone to bone are called:
   a. mycocardia.
   b. tendons.
   c. ligaments.
   d. tendrils.

36. Which of the following forms a socket for a ball and socket joint?
   a. Clavicle.
   b. Patella.
   c. Sternum.
   d. Scapula.

37. The shoulder girdle forms the upper part of the thorax. It is made up of:
   a. the carpals and the scapulae.
   b. the clavicles and the phalanges.
   c. the scapulae and the metacarpals.
   d. the clavicles and the scapulae.

38. The last 2 pairs of ribs are called "floating" ribs because they:
   a. connect directly to the sternum.
   b. connect to the sternum by means of the same cartilage as the 2 pairs of ribs above.
   c. are not connected to the sternum.
   d. are connected neither to the sternum nor the vertebrae.

39. In addition to allowing for motion, skeletal muscles also provide:
   a. body heat.
   b. transportation of oxygen.
   c. transportation of carbon dioxide.
   d. body cooling.

40. The type of muscle tissue found in the gastrointestinal tract is:
   a. smooth muscle tissue.
   b. voluntary muscle.
   c. cardiac muscle tissue.
   d. striated muscle tissue.

Answers to Review Questions

1: b. Voluntary (skeletal) muscle moves bones.

2: b. The insertion of a muscle is on the bone it flexes or extends.

3: d. The tibia articulates with the femur to form the knee joint.

4: c. The fourth through tenth pairs of ribs are most frequently fractured. The first three pairs are protected by the shoulder girdle.

5: a. The radius articulates with the humerus.

6: c. The sternum, or breastbone, joins the ribs at the front of the chest.

7: b. The mandible is the lower jaw.

8: b. A dislocation occurs at a joint.

9: b. Synovial fluid lubricates the bone ends at a joint.

10: a. Involuntary muscles contract without our conscious control.

11: a. Muscle tissue is unique because it can contract.

12: b. The biceps is an example of voluntary muscle.

13: c. The diaphragm is *both* a voluntary and an involuntary muscle.

14: d. Skeletal muscles are voluntary.

15: c. The knee is a hinge joint.

16: c. Antagonistic muscles work in opposition to each other—one contracts to extend a bone, a second contracts to flex it.

17: c. The clavicles can be fractured but are not usually dislocated.

18: d. The muscles lining the intestines are involuntary.

19: d. Ball and socket joints allow for motion in all directions.

20: b. Articular cartilage forms the end of a bone.

21: d. These patients should be given deliberate, careful treatment and transported to prevent further injury.

22: a. The femurs are the largest, heaviest bones in the body.

23: a. Of these choices, the cranium is the only fused joint.

24: c. The hip is a ball and socket joint.

25: b. The individual vertebrae are classified as irregular bones.

26: b. Three pairs of bones, the ischium, ilium, and pubis, fuse in an adult to form the pelvic bone.

27: d. The tibia and fibula make up the lower leg.

28: a. The radius and ulna make up the lower arm.

29: c. The rib cage is made up of 12 pairs of ribs.

30: d. All of these are functions of the skeletal system.

31: b. Approximately 200 bones make up the human skeleton.

32: c. The xiphoid process is the cartilaginous structure at the inferior end of the sternum.

33: c. Muscles *cannot* push a bone.

34: a. Sprains affect ligaments and usually occur at joints.

35: c. Ligaments attach bone to bone; tendons attach muscle to bone.

36: d. The scapula forms a socket for the ball and socket joint at the shoulder.

37: d. The scapulae and clavicles form the shoulder girdle.

38: c. They are called "floating ribs" because they do *not* connect to the sternum.

39: a. Skeletal muscles produce body heat. Heat is released by the chemical reactions that cause skeletal muscles to contract.

40: a. Smooth muscle tissue lines the walls of the gastrointestinal tract.

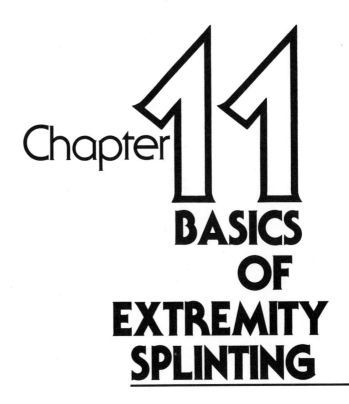

Chapter **11**
**BASICS
OF
EXTREMITY
SPLINTING**

Comprehensive Questions

1. What is the purpose of a splint?

2. List and describe the various types of extremity splints available and discuss the uses, advantages, and disadvantages of each.

3. Why should no splint be applied until a full body survey has been conducted.

4. Explain the principle behind the bone-joint-bone and joint-bone-joint rules of splinting.

5. Why is it necessary for splinted extremities to be immobilized further? How is this immobilization most commonly achieved?

6. Explain the reasoning behind this statement: "You must conform the splint to the needs of the body, not conform the body part to the limits of the splint."

7. What are the accepted general practices regarding the straightening of an injured limb before splinting as opposed to splinting it in the position found? What is the reasoning behind these practices?

8. Why must all major wounds be splinted regardless of whether there has been a fracture?

9. Why is it important to check circulation and neurological function distal to the injury before and after splinting?

Performance Skills

1. Assess and splint a suspected fracture or dislocation of the:
   - a. clavicle.
   - b. scapula.
   - c. humerus.
   - d. elbow.
   - e. radius or ulna.
   - f. wrist.
   - g. hand.
   - h. finger.
   - i. pelvis or hip.
   - j. knee.
   - k. tibia or fibula.
   - l. ankle.
   - m. foot.
   - n. ribs.

2. Properly apply:
   - a. wood splint.
   - b. ladder splint.
   - c. air splint.
   - d. cardboard splint.
   - e. sling and swathe.

Reference Data

1.

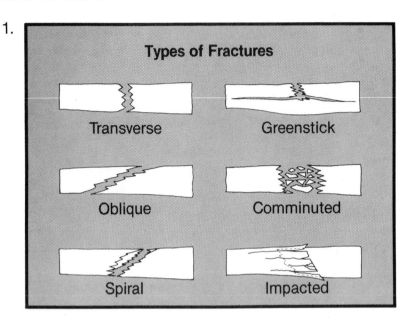

Types of Fractures

Transverse   Greenstick

Oblique   Comminuted

Spiral   Impacted

2. **General rules for splinting**
   a. Clothing should be cut away from all fractures or dislocations before splinting.
   b. The quality of circulation and neurological function distal to the injury should be checked both before and after splinting.
   c. No splint should be applied until all possible fractures have been located.
   d. Severely angulated long bone fractures should be straightened with gentle traction before splinting.
   e. Dislocations or fractures of the shoulder or elbow should not be straightened unless circulation is impaired.
   f. Dislocations of the hip should not be straightened. Fractures of the hip may be straightened for the application of a traction splint.
   g. Dislocations or fractures of the wrist, ankle, or knee should be gently straightened, but not forced before splinting.
   h. Any open wound must be covered with a dressing.
   i. Bone ends or fragments should not be pushed back beneath the skin.
   j. Splinting of a bone should immobilize the joints above and below it. Splinting of a joint should immobilize the bones above and below it.
   k. All splints should be thoroughly padded.
   l. All fractures and dislocations should be splinted before moving the patient, except in extreme cases.
   m. After splinting, splinted extremities should be immobilized.

Review Questions

Select the correct answer for each of the following questions. There is only *one* correct answer for each.

1. A fractured elbow should be immobilized in the position in which it is found because movement may cause:
    a. further fracture.
    b. radial fracture.
    c. damage to nerves and blood vessels.
    d. a dislocation.

2. Applying traction to a fractured limb is best defined as:
    a. the stabilization of a broken bone.
    b. the realignment of bone ends.
    c. the stretching of a broken limb until the broken ends slip into place.
    d. the application of tension to a broken limb.

3. Which of the following statements about fractures is the most accurate?
    a. No fracture presents a threat to life.
    b. Few fractures present a threat to life.
    c. Many fractures present a threat to life.
    d. All fractures present a threat to life.

4. You should inflate an air splint to a point where:
    a. the wrinkles in the splint are about to disappear.
    b. the wrinkles in the splint have just disappeared.
    c. the splint can be slightly dented with thumb pressure.
    d. the splint cannot be dented with thumb pressure.

5. Which of the following splints should *not* be used when treating an open fracture where bone ends or fragments are protruding?
    a. Padded wooden boards.
    b. Padded wire or ladder splints.
    c. Inflatable splints.
    d. Cardboard splints.

6. An injury in which ligaments are stretched or torn, usually from motion forcing them beyond the normal range of the joint, is called a:
    a. fracture.
    b. dislocation.
    c. sprain.
    d. strain.

7. When splinting an open fracture, you should:
   a. splint prior to dressing the wound.
   b. dress the wound prior to splinting.
   c. allow the material that secures the splint to serve as a dressing.
   d. avoid dressing the wound except in very minor compound fractures.

8. Which of the following are signs of a closed fracture?
   a. Deformity.
   b. Point tenderness.
   c. Swelling and/or discoloration.
   d. All of the above.

9. Which of the following types of fractures is most often found in infants and children?
   a. Greenstick.
   b. Open.
   c. Oblique.
   d. Spiral.

10. The patient with a fractured clavicle typically sits or stands with the shoulder of the:
    a. injured side bent backward.
    b. uninjured side bent forward.
    c. uninjured side bent backward.
    d. injured side bent forward.

11. Which of the following can indicate the presence of a fractured pelvis?
    a. Point tenderness over pelvis.
    b. Crepitus or grating.
    c. Pain with movement of one or both legs.
    d. All of the above.

12. When treating a patient with a "silver fork" fracture of the wrist, which of the following splints should not be used by the attending EMTs?
    a. Padded wooden board.
    b. Padded ladder splint.
    c. Inflatable splint.
    d. Padded cardboard splint.

13. When treating a patient with a suspected fracture of the forearm, which of the following should also be immobilized by the attending EMTs?
    a. Wrist.
    b. Elbow.
    c. Shoulder.
    d. All of the above.

14. When treating a patient with a suspected fracture of the lower leg, which of the following should also be immobilized?
    a. Ankle and foot.
    b. Knee and femur.
    c. Hip.
    d. All of the above.

15. You should treat a suspected sprain or strain:
    a. by applying cold applications.
    b. by applying an elastic bandage loosely.
    c. as a minor injury.
    d. as you would a fracture.

16. A dislocation is considered a high priority injury when:
    a. the dislocation is of the hip.
    b. there is loss of the distal pulse and/or sensation.
    c. there is severe angulation of the joint.
    d. the patient is unconscious.

17. To locate a closed fracture in a conscious patient:
    a. ask where the pain is most severe.
    b. look for the area with most swelling.
    c. palpate the bone.
    d. look for discoloration.

18. When treating suspected fractures of the extremities, you should:
    a. move the part to ascertain the extent of the fracture.
    b. splint the part as you find it, whenever possible.
    c. splint first, then control bleeding in open fractures.
    d. move the part across the body for better support.

19. The aims of splinting include all of the following *except*:
    a. reducing open fractures.
    b. preventing damage to nerves and blood vessels.
    c. keeping the bone ends immobile.
    d. preventing the bone ends from piercing the skin.

20. Straighten angulated fractures with the exception of the:
    a. shoulder or elbow.
    b. knee.
    c. wrist or ankle,
    d. all of the above.

21. The most important thing that an EMT should remember about severely angulated fractures is that:
    a. the angulation may cause pinching or cutting of nerves and blood vessels.
    b. the angulation will cause severe pain.
    c. the angulation will make transportation difficult.
    d. the angulation may result in shortening of the limb.

22. After splinting a fractured elbow, the radial pulse of the injured arm becomes very weak and the patient complains of loss of sensation. The EMT should:
    a. transport the patient to the hospital without delay.
    b. unsplint the arm, reposition it, and then resplint it.
    c. position the splinted arm lower than the patient's body.
    d. position the splinted arm higher than the patient's body.

23. When splinting a fractured hand, the hand should:
    a. be covered by the splint on the sides only.
    b. be maintained in the position of function.
    c. not be totally immobilized.
    d. be splinted to the shoulder.

24. The greatest danger in attending to most closed fractures is:
    a. hemorrhage.
    b. danger of opening it.
    c. infection.
    d. shock.

25. To effectively immobilize a fractured clavicle you should apply:
    a. a sling and swathe.
    b. an inflatable splint over the entire arm.
    c. a traction splint to the arm of the injured side.
    d. a rigid splint to the upper arm, then a sling.

26. Fractured patellas are common in car accidents as a result of:
    a. impact of the face against the steering wheel.
    b. impact of the knee against the dashboard.
    c. impact of the elbow against the dashboard.
    d. none of the above.

27. Sprains are injuries where:
    a. the joint is dislocated.
    b. the joint is fractured and the ligaments torn.
    c. the ligaments around the joint are stretched or torn.
    d. the muscles are stretched or torn.

28. To locate possible fractures in an unconscious patient:
    a. palpate the bones of the body carefully without moving the patient.
    b. look for deformity.
    c. look for areas of discoloration.
    d. all of the above.

29. The victim of a shoulder dislocation is found lying on his back. The victim should be transported to the hospital:
    a. after the arm is straightened and splinted.
    b. lying prone with arm hanging of its own weight.
    c. after the arm is placed in a sling and swathe.
    d. with the arm splinted in the position found.

30. Which of the following can be used to splint a midshaft fracture of the humerus?
    a. A short wooden or cardboard splint.
    b. A ladder or wire splint.
    c. The patient's torso.
    d. All of the above.

31. For a suspected pelvic fracture, do all of the following *except*:
    a. immobilization with backboard or stretcher.
    b. traction.
    c. permitting patient to flex his knees.
    d. preventing shock.

32. Fractures of the hip in elderly people:
    a. are common.
    b. may be caused by even a minor fall.
    c. are usually painful.
    d. all of the above.

33. When examining suspected fractures of the extremities, you should:
    a. check the pulse at a non-injured site before splinting.
    b. check the pulse distal to the injury before splinting.
    c. check pulses distal to the injury after splinting.
    d. all of the above.

34. After grasping the limb above and below the fracture site, the EMT should:
    a. slip on a splint.
    b. apply steady traction as the splint is applied.
    c. push back exposed bone ends as the splint is applied.
    d. pull on the bone as the splint is applied.

35. A 53-year-old man leaps from his third floor apartment window to escape a fire. Although he tumbles in the air, he manages to land feet first. You should:
    a. get this man to come over to your ambulance immediately so you can check him.
    b. treat any cuts and burns and transport to the hospital if they are bad enough.
    c. suspect impacted lower extremity fractures and fractures of the spine.
    d. check all burns carefully to be sure no third degree burns have been received.

36. When treating a suspected fracture to a patient's knee, which of the following must also be immobilized?
    a. Hip, femur, tibia/fibula, ankle.
    b. Ankle, tibia/fibula, femur.
    c. Femur and knee.
    d. Knee and tibia/fibula.

37. When treating suspected fractures of the extremities, you should:
    a. elevate the part above the heart.
    b. splint the injured bone and the joints adjacent to it.
    c. return the body to the long, normal configuration.
    d. move the part to ascertain extent of fracture.

38. The best method for splinting a fractured foot is to use:
    a. a ladder splint.
    b. a pillow.
    c. a traction splint.
    d. an air splint.

39. A fracture of the hip is best splinted by:
    a. keeping the leg perfectly straight with a long wood splint.
    b. using an air splint.
    c. placing pillows between the legs and fastening the legs together.
    d. using a sling and swathe.

40. Which of the following is the preferred method for splinting a fractured rib?
    a. Tape firmly around the entire chest.
    b. Place the patient's arm over the fracture site and secure it with swathes.
    c. Lay a short wooden or cardboard splint over the fracture site and secure it with swathes.
    d. Bend a ladder splint to the contour of the chest and secure it with tape.

Answers to Review Questions

1: c. Elbows should be splinted as found to prevent any additional damage to nerves and blood vessels.

2: d. Traction is best defined as the application of tension to a broken limb.

3: b. Few fractures present a threat to life.

4: c. An air or inflatable splint should be inflated until it can be slightly dented with thumb pressure.

5: c. Inflatable splints should *not* be used when bone ends are protruding since the pressure they exert could force the bone ends into the skin.

6: c. A sprain results when ligaments are stretched or torn.

7: b. You should apply a dressing to an open fracture before a splint is applied.

8: d. All of these are signs or indicators of a closed fracture.

9: a. Greenstick fractures are most often found in infants and children.

10: d. The injured side is usually bent forward when a clavicle is fractured.

11: d. All of these are indicators of a fractured pelvis.

12: c. Inflatable splints exert even pressure and may force the wrist to straighten.

13: d. All of these should be immobilized when treating a fracture of the lower arm.

14: d. All of these should be immobilized when treating a fracture of the lower leg.

15: d. Since without x-rays it is impossible to determine that a fracture is *not* present, suspected sprains or strains should be treated as fractures.

16: b. A dislocation is a high priority injury when there is loss of the distal pulse or sensation.

17: a. Ask the patient where the pain is located before you palpate an area or extremity.

18: b. You should splint a part as you find it whenever possible.

19: a. The aims of splinting include all of these except reducing compound fractures.

20: a. Straightening fractures at these joints could damage nerves or blood vessels.

21: a. Angulations may cause pinching or cutting of nerves and blood vessels.

22: b. The proper course of action in this situation would be to unsplint the arm, reposition it, and resplint it.

23: b. The patient's hand should always be maintained in the position of function by having him grasp a roll of gauze.

24: b. The greatest danger is the possibility of causing the fracture to open, or become compound, by mishandling it.

25: a. A sling and swathe is used to immobilize a fractured clavicle.

26: b. Fractures of the patella are often caused by a knee impacting against the dashboard.

27: c. Sprains occur when the ligaments around joints are stretched or torn.

28: d. All of these techniques should be used to locate fractures in an unconscious patient.

29: d. Splint, immobilize, and transport the patient with the limb in the position found.

30: d. All of these objects can be used to splint a fractured humerus.

31: b. Traction is *not* used when a patient has a suspected pelvic fracture.

32: d. All of these statements are correct in regard to hip fractures with elderly people.

33: d. All of these are proper treatment steps when examining a patient for suspected fracture of an extremity.

34: b. Administer steady, gentle traction as the splint is applied.

35: c. In this situation you should suspect impacted fractures of the lower extremities and fractures of the spine.

36: a. The entire extremity including the hip should be immobilized.

37: b. You should splint the bone and the joints adjacent to it. If the joint is injured, you should splint the joint and the bones adjacent to it.

38: b. A pillow will splint the foot and protect it without causing undue pressure.

39: c. A fractured hip is best splinted by placing pillows between the legs and fastening the legs together.

40: b. The arm of the patient's injured side should be placed over the fracture and secured to the chest with swathes.

Practical Applications

Consider how you would act, and why, in the following situations.

1. While walking across the street, a man was struck in the back by a bicyclist. The man complains of a severe pain in the left shoulder. Pain is not increased by normal respirations, but it is aggravated if he tries to move his left arm. Vitals are normal.

2. You arrive at a local school to find a group of children under a tree. They are gathered around a young girl who explains that she fell out of the tree and landed on her right side. She cannot move her right arm and says that she is experiencing great pain in the right shoulder area.

3. A young football player has been injured during a game. When you arrive, his jersey and shoulder pads have been removed. He has pain in his right shoulder and is holding it pitched forward and lower than his left. His vitals are normal. Gentle palpation reveals deformity and pain between the shoulder and the neck of the patient.

4. A young rider fell off his horse during a rodeo. He says, "I just had the wind knocked out of me," but holds the right side of his chest. He appears to be having trouble breathing—his breaths are quick and short as if he is trying not to move. He experiences pain with each inhalation. Otherwise, his vitals are normal.

5. An 18-year-old female was driving a small sports car that was hit on the driver's side by another auto. She complains of severe pain in her hips. Your survey confirms severe pain on compression of the pelvic girdle and no other injuries. Vitals are normal.

6. A 12-year-old boy fell out of a tree while climbing. He complains of pain in his upper left arm. You notice a swollen area just above the elbow. He cries out in pain as you touch his arm. The radial pulse is strong in both wrists. His upper arm is held tightly against his torso.

7. A young man involved in a motorcycle accident complains of severe pain in his left arm. He is found lying on his side holding the injured arm. Your visual survey finds an angulation at the elbow area. The left radial pulse is strong and regular.

8. A woman fell on an icy sidewalk, landing on her hand. When you arrive, she is found sitting inside a store holding her right arm close to her chest. The wrist appears to have the "silver fork" deformity.

9. A 29-year-old housewife has fallen from a stepladder while putting away groceries. She complains of severe pain in her right lower leg. Your survey finds no obvious deformity, but gentle palpation of her leg causes increased pain. The pulse taken below the injury site is strong and regular. Vitals are: pulse, 90; respirations, 20; blood pressure, 110/80.

10. A man was changing his automobile battery when he dropped it on his foot. When you arrive, he is sitting on the ground holding his foot. He is in great pain. His work boot is still on and laced above the ankle. He has suffered no other injury and his vitals are normal.

11. A child playing basketball injures his hand while attempting to catch the ball. You notice deformity in the index finger between the first and second joint. Vitals are normal; there is no other injury.

12. A man's hand was crushed by a machine. When you arrive, he is holding it in a towel. You notice that there is very little bleeding, but there is much deformity and pain. His pulse is 90; respirations are 18; blood pressure is 110/70.

13. A child fell off a swing at a local school. When you arrive, the child is still lying on the ground being comforted by a teacher. The teacher tells you she witnessed the accident and that the child fell on her arm. She adds that she never lost consciousness. The injury site seems to be in the left forearm. The left radial pulse is weaker than the right radial pulse. Other vitals are slightly elevated.

14. A carpenter is found lying on the ground with a severely angulated fracture of the right humerus. The position of the fractured limb makes it impossible to "splint it as it lies" and transport the patient. The right radial pulse is absent. Vitals are: pulse, 80; respirations, 20; blood pressure, 130/80.

15. You find a woman in her late 70s lodged between the wall and a bed. She is unable to move either leg without severe pain. She complains of constant pain in the hip area. She has no airway problem; her pulse is slightly above normal; her pupils are equal.

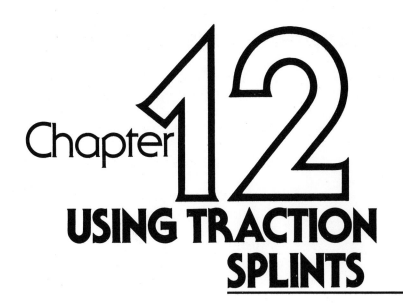

Chapter 12
USING TRACTION SPLINTS

Comprehensive Questions

1. What is the principle of traction and counter traction? How does the traction splint make use of this principle?

2. How is a traction splint different from other splints?

3. Explain how the mechanism of a traction splint works.

4. List the injuries for which use of a traction splint is contraindicated and explain why.

5. Why is the use of a traction splint alone, without a backboard or other supporting device, inappropriate?

6. Why does a fractured femur require traction while many other fractures do not?

7. List the steps for applying a traction splint.

Performance Skills

1. Assess the need for a traction splint.

2. Properly apply the various types of traction splints.

Reference Data

1. Traction splints are generally used to treat fractures of the femur. Some local protocols suggest their use for fractures of the lower leg and hip.

2. The use of traction splints is contraindicated in the following situations:
    a. injuries to the pelvis
    b. injuries to the knee or ankle
    c. when the limb is partially severed
    d. when the patient's systemic condition does not allow time for application

Review Questions

Select the correct answer for each of the following questions. There is only *one* correct answer for each.

1. Unless contraindicated, treat fractures of the femur with:
   a. a ladder splint.
   b. a traction splint.
   c. an inflatable splint.
   d. a long spine board.

2. What is the minimum number of operators necessary to properly apply a traction splint?
   a. 2.
   b. 3.
   c. 4.
   d. 5.

3. Which of the following should not be used as an ankle hitch?
   a. Nylon strap with no shoe or sock.
   b. Leather strap with no shoe or sock.
   c. Web strap with no shoe or sock.
   d. Adhesive tape with no shoe or sock.

4. Applying a traction splint to an arm:
   a. should only be done if there is no injury to the hand, shoulder, or ribs.
   b. should be done using a pediatric leg splint.
   c. should only be done for fractures of the humerus.
   d. should never be done.

5. Which of the following is *not* accomplished by traction splinting?
   a. Counteraction of overriding.
   b. Reducing hemorrhage.
   c. Adequate immobilization of the fractured limb.
   d. Counteraction of muscle spasm.

6. When treating a patient with a suspected fracture of the femur, which of the following must also be immobilized?
   a. Knee and lower leg.
   b. Hip.
   c. Both *a* and *b*.
   d. Neither *a* nor *b*.

7. Which of the following is correct when a patient has a closed fracture of the femur?
   a. Administering oxygen is of little value.
   b. Use direct pressure to control the bleeding.
   c. A tourniquet should be applied above the fracture site.
   d. The patient could go into shock.

8. You should suspect that a patient has fractured a femur when you see the injured leg:
   a. rotated inward and foreshortened.
   b. rotated inward and not shortened.
   c. rotated outward and shortened.
   d. angled backward and not shortened.

9. You should apply longitudinal pull with a traction splint until:
   a. the limb is straightened noticeably.
   b. the patient feels relief.
   c. the bone ends realign.
   d. the fracture is reduced.

10. Which of the following pieces of equipment are required to treat a suspected fracture of the femur?
    a. Traction splint, hitches, and cravats.
    b. Long board and straps or cravats.
    c. Oxygen inhalation.
    d. All of these.

11. In addition to the application of a traction splint, a patient with a suspected fracture of the femur should also be treated for:
    a. anaphylaxis.
    b. shock.
    c. a CVA.
    d. myocardial infarction.

12. Which of the following cannot be used to immobilize a patient with a suspected fractured hip?
    a. Full backboard.
    b. Hare traction splint.
    c. Inflatable splint.
    d. Spit litter.

13. When properly applied, a traction splint will:
    a. stabilize a broken bone.
    b. assist in controlling internal bleeding at the fracture site.
    c. reduce the amount of pain that the patient feels.
    d. all of the above.

14. Of the following, what is the most important reason for the EMT to use a traction splint?
    a. The stabilization of a broken bone.
    b. The reduction of a fracture.
    c. The realignment of bone ends.
    d. The stretching of a broken limb until the broken ends slip back into place.

Answers to Review Questions

1: b. Unless contraindicated, fractures of the femur should be treated with traction splints.

2: a. At least 2 operators are necessary to properly apply a traction splint; 3 operators are preferred.

3: d. Adhesive tape should not be used directly on the skin.

4: d. A traction splint should *not* be applied to an arm.

5: c. The splint will not adequately immobilize the fractured limb. Once the splint is applied, the patient should be placed on a long board to immobilize the pelvis and hip.

6: c. The hip, knee, and lower leg should all be immobilized.

7: d. A patient could lose enough blood into the soft tissues to go into shock.

8: c. The leg generally will rotate outward and be shortened.

9: b. You should apply traction until the patient feels relief.

10: d. All of these will be needed to provide proper emergency care to a patient with a suspected fracture of the femur.

11: b. A patient with a fractured femur should be treated for shock.

12: c. Inflatable splints do not immobilize a hip.

13: d. All of these will be accomplished by the proper use of a traction splint.

14: a. The most important reason for using a traction splint is for the stabilization of a broken bone.

Practical Applications

Consider how you would act, and why, in each of the following situations.

1. A motorcyclist has been struck from the side by an auto. You find him lying on the ground moaning. His face and lips are pale and ashen. There is marked deformity of his left thigh, but there is no break in the skin. Pulse is 120 and weak; respirations are 20; blood pressure is 90/60.

2. A 29-year-old woman was struck by a truck while walking across a street. You find her lying at the side of the street in much pain. She is clutching her left upper leg, but is not having trouble breathing. Your survey indicates deformity and pain mid-thigh. There are no other injuries and no external bleeding. Pulse is 100 and weak; respirations are 24; blood pressure is 80/40.

3. A 10-year-old child fell from a skateboard while going down a steep hill. He has fractured his left femur. Your arrive to find the bone ends protruding through the skin. There is visible bleeding. Pulse is 120 and thready; respirations are 30 and shallow; blood pressure is 60/30.

4. A bicyclist has fallen from his bike and appears to have a fractured right femur. He has marked deformity and pain mid-thigh. His right ankle is bent at an odd angle and he complains of increased pain as you palpate it. Pulse is 100 and regular; respirations are 24; blood pressure is 94/50.

5. A 72-year-old woman fell while getting out of bed. She has pain and deformity in the left femur and also complains of pain in her left hip. The femur break appears to be near the knee. Pulse is 100 and thready; respirations are 24 and shallow; blood pressure is 100/60.

Chapter **13**

IMMOBILIZING NECK AND BACK INJURIES

Comprehensive Questions

1. Describe the anatomy of the spinal column.

2. Why are injuries to the spinal column serious? Why is it important to treat them quickly and carefully?

3. What are the principle signs of a neck or back injury?

4. Why is the mechanism of injury especially important in diagnosing an injury to the neck or back?

5. Describe in sequence and detail the steps which must be taken to immobilize a neck or back injury regardless of what device is being used.

6. What is the purpose of applying hand traction to a patient with suspected neck injury?

7. List the devices available to the EMT for interim immobilization of a sitting patient with suspected neck or back injuries. Describe each one and discuss its advantages, disadvantages, and contraindications.

8. Explain why you must fasten the device to the patient's torso before immobilizing the patient's head to the device.

9. List the devices available to the EMT for full immobilization of a neck or back injury. Describe each one and discuss its advantages, disadvantages, and contraindications.

10. Explain why a split litter is not a good spine immobilization device.

11. What methods are available to the EMT for placing a prone or supine patient with suspected spinal injury onto a long backboard?

12. What additional steps must be taken when transporting a spinal injury patient who has been immobilized on a long backboard?

Performance Skills

1. Assess the need for immobilization of an injury to the neck or back:
    a. in a conscious patient.
    b. in an unconscious patient.

2. Apply cervical traction:
    a. to a sitting patient.
    b. to a supine patient.

3. Determine the proper size extrication (cervical) collar for a patient.

4. Apply an extrication (cervical) collar.

5. Immobilize a sitting patient with an injury to the neck or back with the various types of interim spine immobilization devices.

6. Immobilize to a full backboard a sitting patient that has an interim immobilization device applied.

7. Place a prone or supine patient with an injury to the neck or back on a long board:
    a. with a split litter.
    b. with a body roll.
    c. with a body slide.

8. Immobilize a prone or supine patient with an injury to the neck or back with a full backboard.

9. Immobilize a standing patient with an injury to the neck or back with a full backboard.

Reference Data

1.

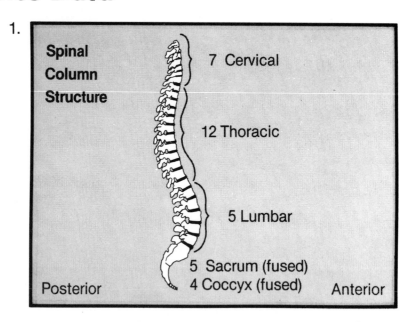

Spinal Column Structure

7 Cervical

12 Thoracic

5 Lumbar

5 Sacrum (fused)
4 Coccyx (fused)

Posterior   Anterior

2.

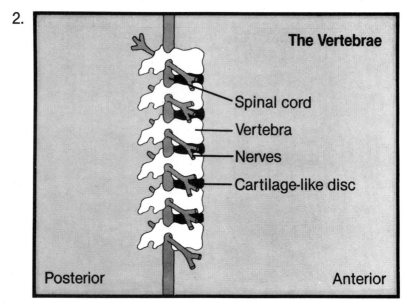

The Vertebrae

Spinal cord

Vertebra

Nerves

Cartilage-like disc

Posterior   Anterior

3.
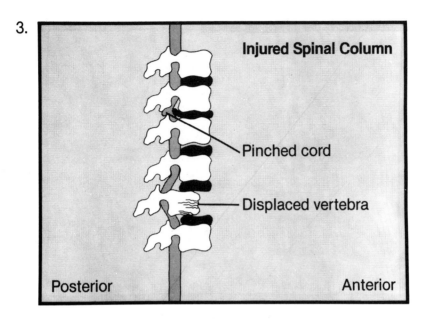

Injured Spinal Column

Pinched cord

Displaced vertebra

Posterior

Anterior

4. **Indicators of spinal injury**
   a. mechanism of injury
   b. other injuries that suggest violent movement and/or sudden stoppage of movement
   c. pain or tenderness at the neck or back
   d. pain when the patient attempts to move
   e. paralysis or numbness to a part of the body
   f. deformity of the neck or back

Review Questions

Select the correct answer for each of the following questions. There is only *one* correct answer for each.

1. How many vertebrae make up the sacral spine?
   a. 4.
   b. 5.
   c. 7.
   d. 12.

2. The vertebrae of the sacral spine:
   a. form hinge joints.
   b. form ball and socket joints.
   c. form gliding joints.
   d. are fused.

3. The spinal column is made up of 33 bones and is divided into:
   a. 3 sections.
   b. 4 sections.
   c. 5 sections.
   d. 6 sections.

4. What is the anatomical name for the first 7 vertebrae of the spinal column?
   a. Sacral.
   b. Lumbar.
   c. Thoracic.
   d. Cervical.

5. Which parts of the spinal column are most commonly injured?
   a. The cervical and thoracic.
   b. The thoracic and lumbar.
   c. The cervical and sacral.
   d. The cervical and lumbar.

6. Which of the following is *not* a usual sign of a spinal cord injury?
   a. Loss of chest wall breathing—only diaphragmatic breathing is evident.
   b. Deformity.
   c. Loss of voluntary motion in the lower extremities.
   d. Loss of voluntary motion in the upper extremities.

7. What signs should you expect if a patient has an injury of the cervical spinal cord?
   a. Chest paralysis and rupture of the diaphragm.
   b. Neck paralysis and rupture of the diaphragm.
   c. Paralysis of the facial and chest muscles.
   d. Paralysis of chest muscles and respiratory difficulty.

8. At the scene of an automobile accident, the driver is found slumped over the steering wheel. He is unconscious and making "snoring" sounds. The victim's neck is in a twisted position. The EMT should carefully:
   a. splint the head in the position it is found.
   b. rotate the head to correct the deformity.
   c. attempt to apply gentle traction and correct the deformity.
   d. hyperextend the neck to correct the deformity.

9. A patient with suspected neck or back injuries can be immobilized on a split litter:
   a. and then placed on the ambulance cot.
   b. and then secured to a full backboard.
   c. instead of a full backboard.
   d. all of the above.

10. The preferred interim device to immobilize a patient with neck or back injuries in a car is the:
    a. short (half) backboard.
    b. build-a-board.
    c. Greene splint.
    d. it is a matter of choice.

11. The lumbar section of the vertebral column is made up of how many bones?
    a. 7.
    b. 12.
    c. 5.
    d. 4.

12. A section of the vertebral column often injured by improperly lifting heavy objects is the:
    a. cervical.
    b. thoracic.
    c. lumbar.
    d. sacral.

13. The cartilaginous discs between vertebrae:
    a. allow for limited motion.
    b. protect the vertebrae from rubbing against each other.
    c. both *a* and *b*.

14. Which section of the spine receives additional bony support?
    a. Cervical.
    b. Thoracic.
    c. Lumbar.
    d. All of the above.

15. The minimum number of EMTs required to log roll a patient is:
    a. 2.
    b. 4.
    c. 6.
    d. 8.

16. A patient involved in a car accident is found unconscious, slumped over the wheel. His ability to feel pain in his hands and feet tells you that:
    a. he has no head or brain injury.
    b. he has no neck or back injury.
    c. his spinal cord is not severed.
    d. there is no need to rush.

17. Assessing for spinal injuries is made easier if the patient is:
    a. conscious and on his back.
    b. conscious and on his side.
    c. unconscious and on his side.
    d. unconscious and on his back.

18. The adjustable seat split litter (build-a-board) is the preferred interim immobilization device when:
    a. the patient has to be moved from a car.
    b. the patient should be immobilized in a sitting position.
    c. the patient's car has deep bucket seats.
    d. the patient is in the back seat of a 4-door sedan.

19. A patient is unconscious, floating face down in a swimming pool. You should:
    a. backboard him in the position he is in, then remove him from the water.
    b. stabilize his neck and back with your hands while you roll him over and secure a patent airway.
    c. turn him over and backboard him.
    d. turn him over, extend his neck to clear the airway, and prepare to float a backboard under him.

20. With the log roll, while 3 EMTs work as a unit to roll the patient, the fourth EMT:
    a. positions the long board.
    b. maintains axial traction.
    c. secures the straps and cravats.
    d. keeps the patient awake.

21. When checking the lower extremities of a conscious patient for paralysis, you should first:
    a. ask the patient to wiggle his toes.
    b. touch the patient's feet and legs and ask him whether he can feel the touch.
    c. ask the patient to raise his legs.
    d. ask the patient to press his foot against your hand.

22. If the mechanism of the accident indicates a possible neck or back injury, the first step after conducting a primary survey is to:
    a. establish an open airway.
    b. immobilize the entire body.
    c. apply and maintain axial traction.
    d. make a complete body survey.

23. The inability of a patient to move his arms and legs following an auto accident should make the EMT suspect an injury to the:
    a. peripheral nerves.
    b. spinal cord in the cervical region.
    c. spinal cord in the thoracic region.
    d. spinal cord in the sacral region.

24. You are alone at the scene of an accident and find a person who is conscious, lying on his back. He cannot move his legs and complains of pain in his back. Which of these should you do first?
    a. Gently raise the patient to a sitting position to see if pain diminishes.
    b. Roll him gently on his stomach; place a pillow or other padding under his head.
    c. Leave him lying on his back; impress upon him that he must not attempt to move; obtain additional help.
    d. Gently lift him on a stretcher and convey him to a place where skilled medical care is available.

25. If a patient must be moved, keep the spinal cord:
    a. well padded.
    b. in traction.
    c. tightly wrapped.
    d. in a straight line.

26. You should treat for a suspected spinal injury:
    a. with an unconscious patient, even if there is no obvious injury.
    b. where there is deformity of the spine.
    c. where there is head injury or paralysis.
    d. all of the above.

27. How many vertebrae make up the thoracic spine?
    a. 7.
    b. 12.
    c. 5.
    d. 4.

28. The spinal cord and nerves that branch from it can be damaged when:
    a. they are pinched between 2 vertebrae.
    b. they are cut or crushed when vertebrae are displaced.
    c. the ligaments supporting the vertebrae are injured.
    d. all of the above.

29. Your patient is seated in the passenger side of the car. You notice the windshield is broken on that side. You should suspect:
    a. pneumothorax.
    b. cervical damage.
    c. eye injury.
    d. cerebrovascular accident.

30. The preferred method to test for paralysis in an unconscious patient is to:
    a. look for dilation of the pupils.
    b. raise the patient's arms and legs and watch for muscular response.
    c. stimulate the soles of the feet and the palms with your fingers or a sharp, pointed object.
    d. any of the above.

31. Which of the following is a common sign of possible neck or spinal cord injury?
    a. Pain at the neck or back.
    b. Inability to move a part of the body.
    c. Loss of sensation in parts of the body.
    d. All of the above.

32. Motor nerves conduct impulses from:
    a. sensory fibers to the brain.
    b. the brain to sensory fibers.
    c. the brain to muscles.
    d. the muscles to the brain.

33. The membranes surrounding the brain and spinal cord are called:
    a. pleurae.
    b. parietal pleura.
    c. meninges.
    d. mesenteries.

34. Which of the following statements accurately describes spinal cord injuries?
    a. All spinal cord injuries can be corrected with surgery.
    b. A severed spinal cord can be surgically repaired.
    c. The injured spinal cord has limited self-healing powers.
    d. A severed spinal cord can rejoin itself.

35. Which of the following is most often injured in automobile accidents producing a "whiplash"?
    a. Cervical spine.
    b. Sacral spine.
    c. Thoracic spine.
    d. Lumbar spine.

Answers to Review Questions

1: b. Five vertebrae fuse in the adult to form the sacral spine.

2: d. The vertebrae of the sacral spine are fused.

3: c. The 33 bones of the spinal column are divided into 5 sections.

4: d. The cervical vertebrae make up the first division of the spinal column.

5: d. The cervical and lumbar sections of the spine are most commonly injured. The thoracic section is protected by the shoulder girdle and ribs, and the sacrum is protected by the pelvic bones.

6: b. While deformity can occur, it is *not* as common as the other indicators listed.

7: d. If the damage is in the cervical area, the nerves controlling respiration may be affected.

8: c. Since there is an airway problem as indicated by the "snoring" sounds, you should attempt to apply gentle traction and correct the deformity.

9: b. A split litter should be used only as an interim device. The patient should be immobilized on a full backboard.

10: a. A short board, or half backboard, is the preferred interim device to immobilize a patient found in a sitting position.

11: c. The lumbar section of the spine is made up of 5 individual vertebrae.

12: c. The lumbar section is often injured when an individual lifts with his back rather than his legs.

13: c. Both of these are functions of the discs between the vertebrae.

14: b. The thoracic section is also supported by the ribs.

15: b. Four EMTs are required to log roll a patient.

16: c. You only know that the cord has *not* been cut; you do not know if the vertebrae are displaced or fractured.

17: a. The assessment of this patient is easier if he is conscious and on his back.

18: b. The build-a-board is the preferred device when the patient should be immobilized in a sitting position.

19: b. You should stabilize the patient's head and neck, roll him as a unit, establish an airway, and begin artificial ventilation as necessary.

20: b. Axial traction must be maintained as the patient is rolled onto the backboard.

21: b. Ask the patient if he can feel the touch of your hands before you ask him to manipulate any part of an extremity.

22: c. Axial traction should be applied and maintained as you complete the patient survey.

23: b. You should suspect a cervical injury if the patient cannot move his arms or legs.

24: c. The course of action described should be followed when you are alone.

25: d. The spinal cord should always be kept in a straight line.

26: d. You should treat a patient for spinal injuries in all of these situations.

27: b. There are 12 vertebrae in the thoracic section of the spinal column.

28: d. All of these conditions can injure or damage the spinal cord.

29: b. You should suspect cervical injury if there is evidence that the patient's head hit the windshield.

30: c. Stimulate the soles and palms and check for a response.

31: d. All of these are signs or indicators of possible spinal cord injury.

32: c. Motor nerves conduct impulses from the brain to muscles.

33: c. The meninges are the membranes that surround the brain and spinal cord.

34: c. The spinal cord has limited ability to heal itself.

35: a. The cervical spine is most often affected when a "whiplash" injury occurs.

Practical Applications

Consider how you would act, and why, in the following situations.

1. You respond to a motor vehicle accident and find the driver standing next to a car with a "starburst" pattern on the windshield. He isn't moving, says his neck hurts, and complains of a tingling sensation in his hands and feet. He tells you that these symptoms came on suddenly as he was giving an accident report to the policeman. Vitals are not alarming.

2. A worker fell from scaffolding and landed on his back. He tells you he can't move. Bystanders tell you he hasn't moved since he fell. Vitals are not alarming.

3. You respond to an auto accident. The only victim is the driver of a large station wagon. He is found sitting behind the wheel, unconscious. There are no obvious injuries. Pulse is 80 and regular; respirations are 20; blood pressure is 110/70. Pupils are dilated and sluggish.

4. Your patient is the driver of a car involved in a motor vehicle accident. She is found behind the wheel, stuporous, with her head tilted towards her left shoulder. The window in the driver's door is cracked. Respirations and other vitals are normal. Pain and resistance are met when you attempt to apply traction and a cervical collar.

5. You respond to a local pool for a diving accident. When you arrive, lifeguards have turned the victim face up and have moved him to shallow water. Witnesses say he struck his head on the side of the pool. He is breathing.

6. A man fell down a flight of stairs. You find him unconscious and prone at the bottom. He shows no reaction to painful stimuli and his vitals are stable. His airway is clear and pupils are unequal.

7. You respond to a motor vehicle accident and find a middle-aged woman lying face down in the back of a four-door sedan. She is unconscious and you suspect cervical injuries. Vitals are normal.

8. A man fell down a flight of stairs. You find him conscious, sitting on the floor and leaning against the wall. He complains that he cannot move his head and feels "tingling" in his legs.

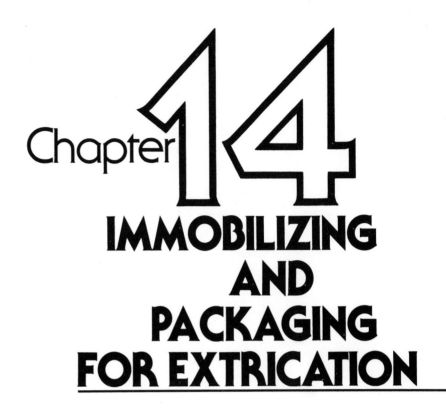

Chapter 14

IMMOBILIZING AND PACKAGING FOR EXTRICATION

Comprehensive Questions

1. Describe the roles and responsibilities of each of the responding emergency services at the scene of an accident.

2. Under what conditions should a victim with suspected neck or back injuries be removed from a vehicle without an interim immobilization device?

3. What are the factors that must be considered when choosing a method of packaging for a patient in need of extrication?

4. What are the factors that must be considered when choosing an extrication route?

5. What should be the EMT's overriding concern at any accident scene?

Performance Skills

Immobilizing and packaging a patient for extrication requires the selection and application of many of the skills acquired at earlier stages of the course. In particular, the skills introduced in the previous chapter, "Immobilizing Neck and Back Injuries," will be very important. In addition, the following performance skills are necessary.

1. Extricate a sitting patient with suspected spinal injury from a damaged vehicle using an interim immobilization device.

2. Without assistance, remove a sitting patient with suspected neck and back injuries from the front seat of a car that may explode.

3. Remove from the front seat of a car a sitting patient with suspected neck and back injuries. The patient's condition is rapidly deteriorating.

4. Immobilize onto a backboard an unconscious patient found lying across the seat of a car.

5. Immobilize onto a backboard an unconscious patient found lying across the floor of a car.

Reference Data

ACCIDENT SCENE RESPONSIBILITIES

1. The **police department** is responsible for control of the accident scene, including:
   a. traffic control and safety from other motor vehicles
   b. crowd control
   c. investigation
   d. re-opening of traffic

2. The **fire service** is responsible for overall scene safety:
   a. to extinguish and protect against fire and explosion
   b. to ensure that rescue and EMS operations can proceed without jeopardy

3. The **rescue squad** is responsible for:
   a. securing the vehicle
   b. gaining access to the victims for the EMTs
   c. opening the vehicle so the patient can be safely extricated

4. The **emergency medical service** is responsible for:
   a. locating all victims
   b. treating patients where they are found
   c. planning extrication route
   d. immobilizing and packaging patients for extrication
   e. removing patients and packaging for transport

ACCIDENT RESPONSE SEQUENCE

1. Fire department makes scene safe from ignition.

2. Rescue squad secures vehicle.

3. Rescue squad provides quick entry.

4. One EMT enters, locates victims, performs primary surveys.

5. All patients completely surveyed.

6. Access for packaging and extrication provided.

7. Patients are treated and packaged.

8. Patients are extricated.

9. Additional treatment provided before transport.

10. Patients monitored and treated during transport.

Review Questions

Select the correct answer for each of the following questions. There is only *one* correct answer for each.

1. The individual who is usually responsible for the safety of all involved at an accident scene is:
    a. the senior police officer.
    b. the senior fire officer.
    c. the senior rescue officer.
    d. the senior EMT.

2. The first responder to most motor vehicle accidents is usually a member of which service?
    a. Police.
    b. Fire.
    c. Rescue.
    d. EMS.

3. The responsibility of investigating the cause of a motor vehicle accident belongs to which service?
    a. Police.
    b. Fire.
    c. Rescue.
    d. EMS.

4. Which service is responsible for gaining access to the patient and providing sufficient space for extrication?
    a. Police.
    b. Fire.
    c. Rescue.
    d. EMS.

5. All unconscious victims of a motor vehicle accident should be suspected of having:
    a. neck injuries.
    b. internal injuries.
    c. pelvic injuries.
    d. all of the above.

6. Which service is responsible for the care and treatment of the victims of a motor vehicle accident?
    a. Fire.
    b. Police.
    c. Rescue.
    d. EMS.

7. When you arrive as the first responder at the scene of a motor vehicle accident, your first concern must be:
   a. to protect the scene from oncoming traffic.
   b. to assure your own safety.
   c. to gain access to the victims.
   d. to secure or stabilize the vehicle involved.

8. When extricating a victim with suspected spinal injury from a vehicle, your choice of the device to be used should be based primarily on:
   a. distance to nearest hospital; fastest device to apply.
   b. type and condition of vehicle; position and medical condition of patient.
   c. medical condition of patient only.
   d. device you are most familiar with using.

Answers to Review Questions

1: b. The safety of all personnel at the scene of an accident is the responsibility of the senior fire officer.

2: a. In most instances, a police officer is the first to arrive at an accident scene.

3: a. The cause of a motor vehicle accident is investigated by the police department.

4: c. It is the role of the rescue service (or the rescue division of a service) to provide access to the victims and enough space for their extrication.

5: d. All of the above are possible. The mechanism of a motor vehicle accident makes these types of injuries likely.

6: d. It is the responsibility of the emergency medical service to treat all victims of a motor vehicle accident.

7: b. The EMT's first concern must always be his own safety.

8: b. When deciding what device you will use to extricate a patient, you must consider the physical situation he is in, as well as his medical priorities.

Practical Applications

Consider how you would act, and why, in each of the following situations.

1. You are the first responder to a motor vehicle accident. As you approach, you see smoke coming from the engine compartment, and one victim slumped over the wheel.

2. You arrive at a motor vehicle accident as chief of an ambulance crew of 3 EMTs. The accident involves 2 cars and 6 people. Police, fire, and rescue services are already on the scene and functioning.

3. You arrive alone as the first responder to a motor vehicle accident. The one vehicle involved seems safe from ignition or further accident. One victim remains in the car, apparently trapped, and two others are lying on the ground nearby.

Chapter 15
INJURIES OF THE HEAD, EYE, MOUTH, AND FACE

Comprehensive Questions

1. Describe the clinical picture associated with a head or brain injury.

2. Explain why even minor bleeding within the skull creates a serious medical condition.

3. What does the appearance of cerebrospinal fluid in the ears or nose indicate about the condition of the head?

4. Describe the anatomy of the eye.

5. Discuss this statement: "Management of facial injuries centers on management of the airway."

Performance Skills

The treatment of injuries of the head, eye, mouth, and face requires the proper selection and application of various skills acquired in earlier stages of the course. In addition, the following performance skills, not previously introduced, will be necessary.

1. Treat a patient for:
   a. a foreign body in the eye.
   b. an object impaled in the eye.
   c. chemical or thermal burns to the eyes, or burns caused by light.
   d. an avulsed eye.
   e. blunt injury to the eye.
   f. lacerations of the eyelids or orbits.

2. Treat a patient for a laceration penetrating through the cheek.

3. Treat a patient for a lacerated artery or vein in the neck.

4. Treat a patient for an object impaled in the cheek, neck, or skull.

5. Assess and treat a patient for suspected facial fractures.

6. Assess and treat a patient for a suspected fracture of the mandible (lower jaw).

7. Assess and treat a patient for a suspected skull fracture.

Reference Data

1. **Indicators of head or brain injury** (*all* of these indicators are not commonly found in any one patient)
   a. deformity or damage to the skull
   b. unresponsive or unequal pupils
   c. double vision
   d. eyes that do not focus or track properly
   e. extreme lethargy or sleepiness
   f. loss of consciousness or deep coma
   g. nausea and vomiting
   h. convulsions
   i. inappropriate or decerebrate reaction to painful stimuli; or lack of reaction
   j. a slow or decreasing pulse rate with an elevated or increasing blood pressure
   k. bleeding or loss of cerebrospinal fluid from the ears, nose, or both
   l. discoloration of tissues under the eyes and behind the ears

2.

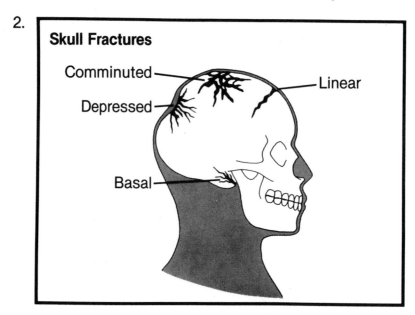

Skull Fractures

Comminuted

Depressed

Linear

Basal

3.

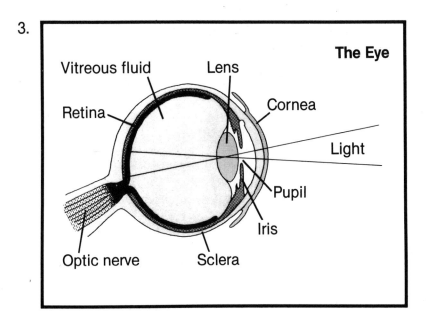

Review Questions

Select the correct answer for each of the following questions. There is only *one* correct answer for each.

1. Which is the best way to control bleeding from a neck artery?
   a. Direct finger pressure.
   b. Tourniquet.
   c. Pressure dressings.
   d. Multi-trauma dressings.

2. The indicators of a head injury include all of the following *except*:
   a. blood and/or clear or cloudy fluid coming from ear or nose.
   b. ecchymosis of the soft tissue under the eye.
   c. "pinpoint" size pupils.
   d. eyes that do not operate together.

3. The iris of the eye:
   a. transmits nerve impulses to the brain.
   b. is the white portion.
   c. regulates the amount of light that enters.
   d. focuses the light on the retina.

4. The globe-like shape of the eye is maintained by the:
   a. vitreous humor.
   b. muscles and ligaments.
   c. iris.
   d. retina.

5. Serious head injury is most often accompanied by:
   a. higher than normal BP and slower than normal pulse.
   b. lower than normal BP and slower than normal pulse.
   c. higher than normal BP and higher than normal pulse.
   d. lower than normal BP and higher than normal pulse.

6. Of the problems listed below, which should the EMT consider when developing a course of treatment for severe facial injuries?
   a. The patient may have received a fractured skull.
   b. The patient may have brain damage.
   c. A neck injury may have been produced by the mechanism of injury.
   d. All of the above.

7. The clear structure of the eye in front of the iris is the:
   a. cornea.
   b. lens.
   c. cilia.
   d. sclera.

8. Which of the following may cause a serious breathing problem in a patient with a facial injury?
    a. Blood clots and loose teeth in the pharynx.
    b. Unconsciousness, with the head flexed forward.
    c. Brain injury.
    d. All of the above.

9. A 45-year-old male appears to have a depressed skull fracture. The EMT should:
    a. bandage the wound without any pressure and elevate the patient's head slightly.
    b. not dress the wound at all.
    c. apply bandages with firm pressure.
    d. bandage the wound without any pressure and lower the patient's head slightly.

10. Surveying an accident victim, you find bleeding from the ears and discoloration under the eyes. What do these signs indicate?
    a. Cerebrovascular accident.
    b. Concussion.
    c. Fractured skull.
    d. Cerebral thrombosis.

11. The first step in treating a patient with a head injury is to:
    a. control bleeding.
    b. establish and maintain an airway.
    c. check for and stabilize any neck injuries.
    d. immobilize the patient's head.

12. When a patient has a foreign object impaled in the globe of his eye, the EMT should:
    a. remove the object, close the eyelid gently, and bandage the eye with a snug pressure dressing.
    b. place a loose dressing over the object and bandage the uninjured eye.
    c. apply a thick dressing and secure a protective cone over the impaled object, leaving the uninjured eye unbandaged.
    d. apply a thick dressing and secure a protective cone over the impaled object; also bandage the uninjured eye.

13. Fracture of the larynx is most likely when which of the following is injured?
    a. The sternum.
    b. The face.
    c. The neck.
    d. The clavicle.

14. If a portion of the ear, scalp, or nose is completely avulsed, it should be:
    a. left alone and not disturbed.
    b. repositioned on the injury site with tape.
    c. placed in a container of water and transported to the hospital with the patient.
    d. placed on a sterile dressing, moistened with sterile saline, kept cold, and transported to the hospital with the patient.

15. When treating a patient with an injury to the eye, both the injured and uninjured eye should be covered to reduce:
    a. collateral circulation.
    b. sympathetic movement.
    c. fear and anxiety.
    d. tearing and paradoxical movement.

16. Cerebrospinal fluid:
    a. provides nourishment for some brain cells.
    b. acts as a shock absorber for the brain and spinal cord.
    c. is found between the tissues that surround the brain and cord.
    d. all of the above.

17. A small foreign body may be removed from a patient's eye by:
    a. his own tears.
    b. irrigating the eye with sterile water or saline.
    c. carefully using a wet sterile applicator.
    d. all of these.

18. How does maintenance of an airway for a patient with a head injury differ from the usual technique?
    a. The mouth is not swept clear at first.
    b. The head injury is given priority over airway maintenance.
    c. Hyperextension of the head is contraindicated.
    d. The jaw is not lifted.

19. A little boy sprayed oven cleaner in his eyes. You should:
    a. rush him to the hospital.
    b. have someone call the poison control center while you bandage his eyes.
    c. pour tap water in his eyes for 20 minutes.
    d. immediately neutralize with lemon juice or vinegar, then transport to the hospital.

20. If cerebrospinal fluid is present in the ear or nose, the EMT should:
    a. pack the ears, and allow the nose to drain.
    b. do nothing.
    c. cover the openings with a loose dressing.
    d. cover the openings with a firm dressing.

21. If the patient is unconscious, the EMT can suspect brain damage if there has been a head injury and the pupils of the eyes are:
    a. equal and reactive.
    b. constricted.
    c. paradoxical.
    d. unequal.

22. A sliver of glass is impaled in the patient's cheek and extends into the oral cavity. Proper treatment includes:
    a. removing the glass sliver, and holding gauze against the inside and outside of the cheek to control bleeding.
    b. not removing the glass sliver, just holding gauze against the inside and outside of the cheek.
    c. tilting the head to the uninjured side and slightly lowering the cheek and mouth without flexing the head.

23. If you are treating an adult patient for a head injury and he goes into shock, you should suspect:
    a. brain damage.
    b. concussion.
    c. cerebral edema.
    d. another serious injury.

24. During a karate class a student is struck in the throat by his partner's fist and falls to the ground. When the EMT arrives, he should first determine:
    a. if the trachea is fractured.
    b. if the air is escaping into the soft tissue of the neck.
    c. if there is a strong carotid pulse.
    d. if there is a patent airway.

25. If a patient became unconscious immediately after an accident, but has since regained consciousness, he has probably suffered:
    a. laceration.
    b. stroke.
    c. linear skull fracture.
    d. concussion or epidural hematoma.

26. Meninges are tissues that:
    a. surround and protect the brain.
    b. connect the intestines to the abdominal wall.
    c. surround the lungs.
    d. protect cardiac muscle.

27. The spinal cord is:
    a. a separate organ, detached from the brain.
    b. a continuation of the brain.
    c. an independent organ, connected to the brain by muscle.
    d. an independent organ, attached to the brain by vertebrae.

28. The brain is protected by:
    a. the bones of the cranium.
    b. cerebrospinal fluid.
    c. 3 layers of specialized tissue.
    d. all of the above.

29. The brain can be described as a:
    a. semisolid, fairly dry organ, richly supplied with blood.
    b. very firm, moist organ, richly supplied with blood.
    c. semisolid and moist organ, richly supplied with blood.
    d. firm and fairly dry organ, richly supplied with blood.

30. Because the skin of the face and scalp contains many blood vessels, it is said to be very:
    a. muscular.
    b. epidermal.
    c. cervical.
    d. vascular.

31. When the patient has a bleeding head wound, the EMT should:
    a. apply a snug pressure bandage.
    b. apply a loose sterile dressing to aid the clotting process.
    c. apply pressure to the subclavian artery.
    d. lightly pack the wound with sterile dressings.

32. When a foreign object is impaled in the skull, the EMT should:
    a. not remove the object, but stabilize it in place.
    b. remove the object and apply a loose sterile dressing.
    c. not remove the object unless it will hinder transportation.
    d. remove the object and pack the wound with sterile pads.

33. Because of possible airway difficulty associated with facial injuries, the unconscious patient should be transported:
    a. on his side.
    b. in a sitting position with his head between his legs.
    c. in a sitting position with his head tilted backward.
    d. lying on his back.

34. A laceration of the eyelid may appear to be very serious. The patient's sight will probably not be lost as long as which of the following is not damaged?
    a. Superior lacrimal gland.
    b. Globe.
    c. Conjunctiva.
    d. Lacrimal duct.

35. The brain may swell when it is injured. This is serious because:
    a. pressure on the brain will cause a hemorrhage.
    b. the swelling may travel to the spinal cord.
    c. there is little room for expansion within the skull.
    d. it is difficult to drain the fluid from the skull.

36. Fractures of the facial bones are dangerous because:
    a. associated bleeding is not easily stopped.
    b. they are not easily repaired.
    c. they may cause airway obstruction.
    d. they generally cause permanent scarring.

37. Which of the following are important signs of head injury where no obvious wounds are present?
    a. Bloody, or a clear fluid, draining from the ear and/or the nose.
    b. Discoloration of soft tissue under the eyes.
    c. Unequal pupils.
    d. All of the above.

Answers to Review Questions

1: a. Applying direct finger pressure is the best way to control bleeding from a lacerated artery in the neck.

2: c. All of these are indicators of a head injury except the presence of "pinpoint" pupils. With a head injury, a patient may exhibit unequal pupils.

3: c. The iris regulates the amount of light that enters the eye.

4: a. The vitreous humor gives the eye its globe-like shape.

5: a. Hypertension (high blood pressure), and bradycardia (slow pulse rate) are indicators of a head injury.

6: d. All of these may be associated with severe facial injuries.

7: a. The cornea is the clear structure in front of the iris.

8: d. All of these conditions can cause breathing problems in a patient with facial injuries.

9: a. A depressed skull fracture should be bandaged with no pressure and the patient's head elevated.

10: c. These are signs or indicators of a fractured skull.

11: b. Establishing and maintaining an airway are the highest priorities of treatment.

12: d. The injured eye and impaled object should be treated with dressings and a cup or protective cone. The uninjured eye should be covered to reduce sympathetic motion.

13: c. Blunt injury to the front of the neck would most likely fracture the larynx.

14: d. A completely avulsed part should be placed on a sterile dressing, moistened with sterile saline, kept cold, and transported with the patient.

15: b. Both the injured and uninjured eye should be covered to reduce sympathetic movement.

16: d. All of these describe the functions of cerebrospinal fluid.

17: d. All of these are accepted emergency medical treatment for removing a small foreign body from a patient's eye.

18: c. Hyperextension of the head is contraindicated with a patient having a head injury because there may be an associated neck injury.

19: c. The patient's eyes should be flushed continuously for about 20 minutes to remove all traces of the caustic agent.

20: c. A loose dressing should be applied if cerebrospinal fluid is draining.

21: d. Unequal pupils in an unconscious patient are an indicator of a head injury.

22: a. An object impaled in a patient's cheek should be removed if it can cause further injury, or if it interferes with the airway.

23: d. You should look for another serious injury. Low blood pressure or shock rarely result from brain damage.

24: d. The EMT should first determine if there is spontaneous respiration and adequate air exchange.

25: d. The patient has had a concussion or epidural hematoma if he lost, and then regained, consciousness.

26: a. Meninges are tissues that surround and protect the brain.

27: b. The spinal cord is a continuation of the brain.

28: d. All of these protect the brain.

29: c. The brain is a semisolid, moist organ that is richly supplied with blood.

30: d. The term "vascular" means relating to or containing blood vessels.

31: a. A snug pressure bandage should be applied.

32: a. An impaled object, except in the cheek, should not be removed but should be stabilized in place.

33: a. The unconscious patient should be transported on his side to aid in the management of his airway.

34: b. The patient's sight will probably not be lost unless the globe is also damaged.

35: c. Swelling of the brain is dangerous because there is little room for expansion within the skull, thus compressing the brain tissue.

36: c. Fractures of the facial bones may cause the patient's airway to be obstructed.

37: d. All of these are indicators of a head injury in the absence of obvious trauma.

Practical Applications

Consider how you would act, and why, in the following situations.

1. A middle-aged man who was involved in a knife fight has been cut across his neck. A deep wound is bleeding severely. His pulse is rapid and thready.

2. A woman passenger was struck by flying debris during an auto accident. A piece of glass has penetrated her cheek and protrudes into the mouth. There are no other injuries and vitals are normal.

3. An elderly man fell in the bathroom breaking the mirror and is found with a laceration of his left eyelid. The bleeding has stopped by the time you arrive. The laceration is 1 inch long and fairly wide. It appears to widen each time the victim blinks his eye. Vitals are normal, and the victim states he did not lose consciousness.

4. A young man's right ear has been cut by a knife. The wound is bleeding freely when you arrive. Your survey locates a flap of loose skin. Vitals are normal and there are no other injuries.

5. The victim of an auto accident does not complain of injury, but his face and hair are blood-soaked. Your survey indicates a scalp laceration that is bleeding freely. There are no other apparent injuries. Vitals are normal.

6. A fan at a baseball game has been struck on the head by a foul ball. When you arrive at the first aid station, the patient is sitting, holding an ice pack over his left eye, and complaining of a headache. You remove the ice pack and see that the eye has swollen shut. The area around the eye is beginning to discolor.

7. You find an unconscious man "snoring" at the bottom of a flight of stairs about 10 minutes after he fell. You palpate his head and feel a depressed area just above his hair line. Your survey finds no other injuries. His pupils are unequal. Pulse is 60; respirations are 18; blood pressure is 170/110.

8. A young boy was playing football with friends. He was tackled and landed face first on the head of another child. He has a bloody nose that won't stop bleeding. There is pain and swelling evident at the bridge of the nose. He tells you he never passed out and his vision is not blurred. Pulse is 100; other vitals are normal, although he is frightened. The other child is unhurt.

9. While playing in a school soccer game, a 12-year-old boy receives a crushing blow to the facial area. When you arrive at the scene, he

is bleeding profusely from the nose. He also complains of severe headache. Your survey of the patient's eyes reveals double vision and sluggish tracking ability.

10. A young boxer complains of severe pain in his lower jaw. He can't talk because of the pain. You see no deformity, but your attempts to palpate his jaw cause increased pain. All vitals are normal.

11. A woman has called you because she has a piece of dirt in her eye. She tells you that her eye has been tearing for 30 minutes, but that she can still feel the particle.

14. The patient is a victim of a motor vehicle accident. He is confused and moaning behind the wheel of the car. Your survey indicates no apparent injuries. No history is available. Blood pressure is 130/90; respirations are 14; pulse is 70.

15. A young man has been assaulted and is bleeding from the mouth. He is found holding his mouth and has several broken teeth wrapped in a tissue. He says he did not lose consciousness and only his mouth hurts. Vital signs are normal.

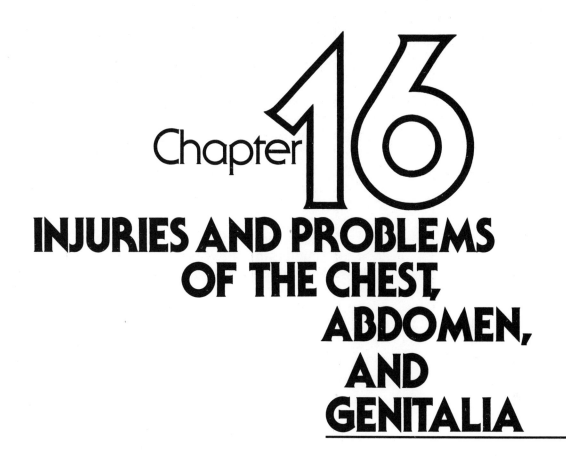

Chapter **16**

INJURIES AND PROBLEMS OF THE CHEST, ABDOMEN, AND GENITALIA

Comprehensive Questions

1. Under what conditions should a thorough examination of the chest be given? What should it include?

2. What is a tension pneumothorax? Describe the process by which a tension pneumothorax creates a progressively more life-threatening condition.

3. What is a sucking chest wound? Why is an occlusive dressing the indicated treatment?

4. What is a flail chest? Explain how the paradoxical motion of the flail segment compromises adequate ventilation.

5. List and describe the serious chest problems that can occur spontaneously without trauma. Describe the clinical picture.

6. What is traumatic asphyxia? Why does a victim exhibit cyanosis of the head and neck?

7. Under what conditions should a thorough examination of the abdomen be given? What should it include?

8. Discuss the possible causes of an acute abdomen and how each causes its clinical picture to develop.

9. How do you control bleeding of the female genitalia?

10. Name the organs which lie within the abdomen and the quadrant in which each is located. Which are hollow organs? Which are solid?

Performance Skills

The treatment of injuries of the chest, abdomen, and genitalia requires the informed selection and specialized application of various skills acquired at earlier stages of the course. The primary new skill required is the ability to recognize the different conditions that may present themselves, and select the proper treatment.

In addition, the following performance skills, not previously introduced, will be necessary.

1. Treat a patient with a sucking chest wound using an occlusive dressing.

2. Treat a patient with a flail chest by properly splinting the injury.

3. Treat a patient with an evisceration of the abdomen.

4. Treat a patient with an acute abdomen.

5. Treat a patient with vaginal bleeding.

Reference Data

1. **Indicators of chest injury**
   a. abnormal respiratory rate
   b. abnormal or paradoxical movement of the chest or rib cage
   c. dyspnea or cyanosis
   d. local pain, or pain aggravated by breathing
   e. coughing blood, or the presence of pink, frothy sputum.
   f. diaphragmatic breathing.

2. **Common chest injuries**
   a. **flail chest:** fracture of 3 or more ribs, each in 2 places; or fracture of several ribs and the sternum.

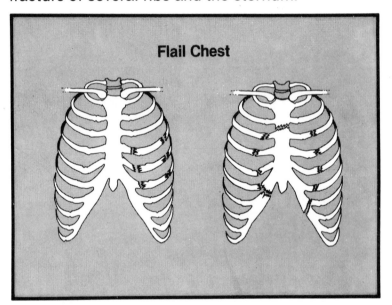

Flail Chest

b. **simple pneumothorax:** accumulation of air in the pleural space; from the exterior through a sucking chest wound, or from the lung due to rupture. Note: trachea may tilt toward the injured side.

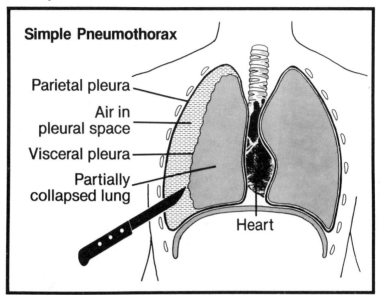

c. **tension pneumothorax:** leakage of air into pleural space with no means of exit. Note: trachea may tilt away from affected side.

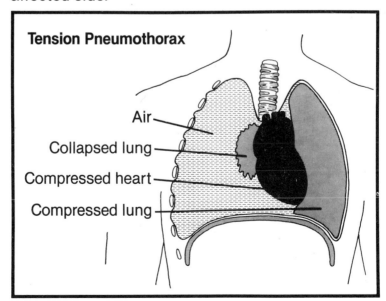

d. **hemothorax:** presence of blood in the pleural cavity. Note: trachea may tilt away from the affected side. May occur in conjunction with pneumothorax (hemopneumothorax).

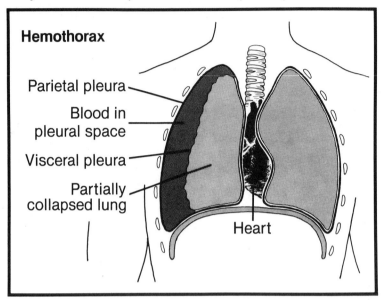

e. **traumatic asphyxia:** severe compression of the chest causes blood to be forced back into the neck veins and subcutaneous bleeding into the tissues of the neck and upper chest.

3. **Signs and symptoms of the acute abdomen**
   a. local or diffuse abdominal pain
   b. local or diffuse abdominal tenderness
   c. a tense, guarded abdomen
   d. elevated pulse rate
   e. low blood pressure
   f. rapid, shallow breathing
   g. patient lies still, not wanting to move

4. **Quadrants of the abdomen**
   a. right upper contains: liver, gallbladder, portion of the colon
   b. left upper contains: stomach, spleen, portions of the colon
   c. right lower contains: appendix, cecum, ascending colon
   d. left lower contains: descending colon, sigmoid colon

5.

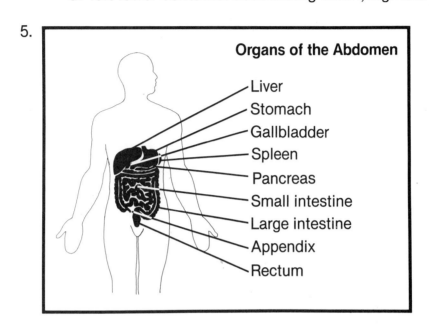

Organs of the Abdomen

Liver
Stomach
Gallbladder
Spleen
Pancreas
Small intestine
Large intestine
Appendix
Rectum

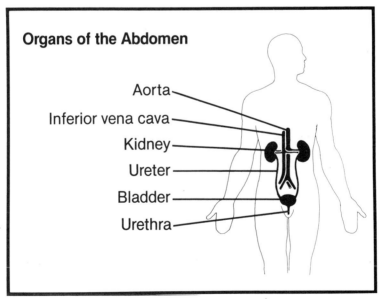

Organs of the Abdomen

Aorta
Inferior vena cava
Kidney
Ureter
Bladder
Urethra

Review Questions

Select the correct answer for each of the following questions. There is only *one* correct answer for each.

1. A person with an abdominal injury should:
   a. not be given anything by mouth.
   b. be allowed to drink small quantitites of fluids, but only upon request.
   c. be given large quantities of saline solution by mouth to combat shock.

2. Into how many sections is the abdomen divided for the purposes of communication, organ location, and diagnosis?
   a. 2.
   b. 4.
   c. 6.
   d. 8.

3. Pain and tenderness in the right upper quadrant of the abdomen, without trauma, often indicates:
   a. ruptured spleen.
   b. appendicitis.
   c. gallbladder disease.
   d. disease of the colon.

4. Pain and tenderness following injury in the left upper quandrant may indicate:
   a. ruptured spleen.
   b. appendicitis.
   c. gallbladder disease.
   d. disease of the colon.

5. The stomach is located in the:
   a. thoracic cavity.
   b. abdominal cavity.
   c. pelvic cavity.
   d. none of these.

6. The liver is located:
   a. under the diaphragm, lying primarily on the right side of the body.
   b. below the stomach, lying primarily in the center of the abdomen.
   c. below the upper abdomen, lying primarily on the right side of the body.
   d. under the diaphragm, lying primarily on the left side of the body.

7. After sealing a sucking chest wound, you note that the patient's ventilation deteriorates, pulse quality weakens, and the blood pressure drops. You should suspect:
    a. tension pneumothorax.
    b. traumatic asphyxia.
    c. spontaneous pneumothorax.
    d. non-traumatic lung injury.

8. A 23-year-old man is suffering from acute onset of shortness of breath, accompanied by pain in his left shoulder which is aggravated by breathing. Lung sounds are clear, although they are somewhat diminished on the left side. You should suspect:
    a. pumonary edema.
    b. spontaneous pneumothorax.
    c. asthma.
    d. acute myocardial infarction.

9. Which of the following is *not* a sign of an acute abdomen?
    a. abdominal pain.
    b. abdominal tenderness.
    c. long, deep breaths.
    d. rapid pulse.

10. Bright red, frothy blood bubbling from the patient's mouth with each exhalation may be an indication of:
    a. lung damage.
    b. abdominal injury.
    c. airway obstruction.
    d. respiratory arrest.

11. Which of the following is the most effective way of ventilating a patient with a flail chest and inadequate ventilation?
    a. Immobilize the chest.
    b. Assist respiration with a bag-valve-mask.
    c. Give mouth-to-mouth ventilation.
    d. Give oxygen by mask.

12. A high school football player received a hard direct blow to the abdomen. Which of the following might indicate the presence of a ruptured spleen?
    a. Vomiting of blood with rapid breathing; rapid pulse.
    b. Rapid, shallow breathing; left upper quadrant pain, decreased blood pressure, and rapid pulse.
    c. Rapid breathing; restlessness; discoloration of abdomen.
    d. Lower right quadrant pain; rapid pulse; nausea; rapid, shallow breathing.

13. A 30-year-old man had been pinned under an automobile that slipped from a jack. Upon arrival, you find the automobile has been removed by the rescue team. The patient displays rapid and shallow breathing, inward movement of the chest wall during inspiration, cyanosis, and hypotension. What is the most likely diagnosis?
    a. Hemothorax.
    b. Ruptured main stem bronchus.
    c. Hemopericardium.
    d. Flail chest.

14. What effect does the accumulation of blood, fluid, or air in the chest cavity have on lung inflation?
    a. Increases it.
    b. Decreases it.
    c. No effect on inflation, but does increase rate of respiration.
    d. No effect on inflation, but does decrease rate of respiration.

15. A patient has been in an auto accident. His lips and tongue are cyanotic. His eyes are bloodshot and bulged, his head and shoulders appear dark blue. He is struggling to breathe. The EMT should treat this patient for:
    a. traumatic asphyxia.
    b. flail chest.
    c. spontaneous pneumothorax.
    d. tension pneumothorax.

16. What does the term "hemothorax" mean?
    a. Air in the chest cavity.
    b. Blood in the chest cavity.
    c. Blood in the airway.
    d. Blood in the pericardial sac.

17. If the abdomen is lacerated and an abdominal organ protrudes, you should:
    a. supply transport as rapidly as possible.
    b. cover it with sterile dressings.
    c. cover it with moist sterile dressings, and keep them moist.
    d. reinsert the protruding organ.

18. You are on your way to care for the victim of a chest injury. Which one of the following conditions would you be unlikely to find when you arrive?
    a. Pneumothorax.
    b. Traumatic asphyxia.
    c. Subcutaneous emphysema.
    d. Evisceration.

19. An organ that lies below the diaphragm and above the left kidney is often ruptured as a result of an abdominal injury. The name of this organ is the:
    a. spleen.
    b. urinary bladder.
    c. gallbladder.
    d. duodenum.

20. Your survey of a multiple-trauma patient finds significant abdominal rigidity. This is suggestive of:
    a. ruptured spleen.
    b. ruptured intestine.
    c. ruptured bladder.
    d. all of the above.

21. The urinary bladder is located in the:
    a. thoracic cavity.
    b. abdominal cavity.
    c. pelvic cavity.
    d. none of these.

22. The stomach:
    a. makes blood.
    b. is a hollow organ in the left upper quadrant.
    c. lies in the pelvis.
    d. stores and concentrates bile.

23. The thoracic cavity contains the:
    a. lungs.
    b. heart and great vessels.
    c. esophagus.
    d. all of the above.

24. Which of the following signs and symptoms will the EMT see in patients with acute appendicitis?
    a. Pain in the lower left quadrant, nausea, fever.
    b. Cramps in the upper right quadrant.
    c. Pain in the upper quadrants, tender, rigid abdomen.
    d. Pain in lower right quadrant, loss of appetite.

25. If an object has become impaled in the patient's abdomen, the EMT should:
    a. remove it if the patient shows signs of going into shock.
    b. not remove it under any conditions.
    c. remove it if intestines and other internal organs are not protruding.
    d. not remove it unless the patient is thrashing about.

26. You are attending a patient with a sucking chest wound and frothy bright red blood at the mouth. After sealing the chest wall, you suspect that the patient is developing tension pneumothorax. What should be your next action?
    a. Apply direct pressure over the wound to stop the bleeding.
    b. Unplug the seal over the chest wound, then reseal it.
    c. Administer positive pressure ventilation immediately.
    d. Administer pure oxygen to aid respiration.

27. Which of the following conditions may be caused by a penetrating chest wound that opens the pleural sac?
    a. Pneumothorax.
    b. Pleurisy.
    c. Pericarditis.
    d. Traumatic asphyxia.

28. In transporting a patient with abdominal injuries, the EMT should place him on the ambulance cot in the:
    a. supine position with his knees flexed.
    b. prone position with his head flexed.
    c. coma position with his head extended.
    d. coma position with his head flexed.

29. The crackling sensation produced by air escaping into surrounding tissues due to an open chest wound is called:
    a. subcutaneous emphysema.
    b. traumatic asphyxia.
    c. flail chest.
    d. pneumothorax.

30. If a patient is vomiting bright red blood or is vomiting blood which has the appearance of "coffee grounds," you should suspect:
    a. punctured lung.
    b. ruptured aorta.
    c. gastro intestinal bleeding.
    d. ruptured spleen.

31. Indicators of injury to the chest include:
    a. localized pain.
    b. pain aggravated by breathing.
    c. dyspnea.
    d. all of the above.

32. Treatment of the patient with an acute abdomen includes:
    a. administering oxygen by inhalator.
    b. preparing for vomiting.
    c. allowing the patient to flex his legs and lie in a comfortable position.
    d. all of the above.

33. Guarding and rigidity of the abdominal muscles are frequently symptoms of:
    a. pneumothorax.
    b. muscular strain.
    c. bleeding or "dumping of the contents" of injured organs into the abdominal cavity.
    d. bleeding ulcer.

34. Which injury would you be most likely to suspect in the driver of an auto if you notice that the steering wheel column of the vehicle is collapsed?
    a. Flail chest.
    b. Fractured femur.
    c. Ruptured kidneys.
    d. Fractured vertebrae.

35. Which of the following abdominal organs is hollow?
    a. Spleen.
    b. Gallbladder.
    c. Pancreas.
    d. Liver.

36. Which of the following abdominal organs is solid?
    a. Kidney.
    b. Urinary bladder.
    c. Appendix.
    d. Cecum.

37. A patient with a flail chest has difficulty breathing because of multiple fractures, and because:
    a. the negative pressure of air in the lungs is reversed.
    b. the chest cavity is reduced, cutting down on the supply of air into the lungs.
    c. the pressure does not change.
    d. the flail part of the chest results in the loss of normal chest movement.

38. Symptoms of traumatic asphyxia are:
    a. head, neck, and shoulders appear dark blue or purple.
    b. the eyes are bloodshot and bulged.
    c. tongue and lips are swollen and cyanotic.
    d. all of the above.

39. A sucking chest wound is a condition in which:
    a. the sternum has collapsed.
    b. the diaphragm has collapsed or ruptured.
    c. the chest cavity has been penetrated by a foreign object and air has entered.
    d. the muscles around the heart have been torn loose.

40. A condition in which a lung collapses and continual air leaks build up pressure within the chest cavity is called:
    a. tension pneumothorax.
    b. flail chest.
    c. subcutaneous emphysema.
    d. traumatic asphyxia.

41. The most effective means of preventing air from entering an opening in the chest wall is:
    a. seal it with an occlusive dressing.
    b. tape it closed.
    c. pack it with thick dressings.
    d. tape a small pillow over the opening.

42. An EMT finds a patient with paradoxical movement of the chest. As the patient breathes, the EMT observes that the loose chest section:
    a. moves in and out with the chest cage.
    b. moves in the opposite direction from the rest of the chest cage.
    c. remains still while the chest cage moves in and out.
    d. changes size as the chest cage moves in and out.

43. When treating bleeding from the female genitalia, *do not:*
    a. apply local compression.
    b. place dressings within the vagina.
    c. treat for shock.
    d. treat other injuries in order of their priority.

44. The treatment to control bleeding from the male genitalia is to:
    a. apply direct pressure if possible.
    b. apply moistened sterile dressings.
    c. transport immediately.
    d. elevate the legs.

45. Injuries to both the male and female genitalia:
    a. are very painful.
    b. are rarely life-threatening.
    c. usually cause great anxiety.
    d. all of the above.

46. Emergency treatment for a direct blow to the scrotum is to:
    a. transport immediately.
    b. apply cold packs.
    c. apply moist sterile dressings.
    d. transport the patient on his stomach.

47. An object impaled in the male or female external genitalia:
    a. should be removed to prevent patient embarrassment.
    b. must be left in place and stabilized.
    c. must be removed before transportation.
    d. is no concern of the EMT.

48. Bleeding can be profuse from both the male and female genitalia. In addition to controlling bleeding, the EMT should:
    a. treat all injuries in order of their priority.
    b. treat for shock.
    c. keep avulsed parts moist and cold.
    d. all of the above.

49. Lacerations, avulsions, or contusions to the external female genitalia should be treated by applying:
    a. moist, sterile, dressings.
    b. local pressure.
    c. a diaper-type bandage to hold dressings in place.
    d. all of the above.

Answers to Review Questions

1: a. This patient should be given nothing by mouth.

2: b. The abdomen is divided into 4 quadrants.

3: c. Tenderness in the right upper quadrant of the abdomen often indicates gallbladder disease.

4: a. Tenderness or pain in the left upper quadrant indicates a possible ruptured spleen.

5: b. The stomach is located in the left upper quadrant of the abdominal cavity.

6: a. The liver lies primarily in the right upper quadrant, under the diaphragm.

7: a. These are signs of a tension pneumothorax.

8: b. These are signs of a spontaneous pneumothorax.

9: c. A patient with an acute abdomen will breathe rapidly and not deeply. Long, deep breaths are painful to this patient.

10: a. This is a sign of damage to a lung.

11: b. The ventilations of a patient with a flail chest should be assisted with the use of a bag-valve-mask.

12: b. These are indicators of a possible ruptured spleen.

13: d. These signs indicate a flail chest.

14: b. The presence of blood, fluid, or air in the chest cavity limits the space available for the lungs to expand, decreasing inflation.

15: a. These signs are indicative of traumatic asphyxia. Sudden compression has forced blood back from the right side of the heart into the veins of the head, neck, and shoulders.

16: b. Hemothorax is the presence of blood in the chest cavity.

17: c. The application of moist sterile dressings is the appropriate treatment for an abdominal evisceration.

18: d. An evisceration is not an injury of the chest.

19: a. The spleen is often ruptured by abdominal injury.

20: d. All of these are possible injuries.

21: c. The urinary bladder lies behind the pubic bone in the pelvis.

22: b. The stomach is a hollow organ in the upper left quadrant.

23: d. All of these organs lie in the thoracic cavity.

24: d. The appendix is located in the lower right quadrant. The appendicitis patient will usually have a loss of appetite, as well as pain, nausea, fever, etc.

25: b. The EMT should never remove an impaled object from the abdomen.

26: b. The chest seal should be removed to allow the air under pressure to escape.

27: a. Pneumothorax may be caused by a penetrating chest wound.

28: a. A patient with abdominal injuries should be transported in a supine position.

29: a. Subcutaneous emphysema is the condition in which air escapes into the tissues of the body.

30: c. These are signs of gastro intestinal bleeding.

31: d. All of these are indicators of injury to the chest.

32: d. These are all aspects of proper care of the patient with an acute abdomen.

33: c. Guarding or rigidity of the abdominal muscles may be caused by internal bleeding or the releasing of the contents of abdominal organs.

34: a. This mechanism of injury would indicate the likelihood of a flail chest.

35: b. The gallbladder is a hollow organ.

36: a. The kidney is a solid organ.

37: d. A flail chest results in the loss of normal chest movement.

38: d. All of these are signs of traumatic asphyxia.

39: c. A sucking chest wound is one in which the chest cavity has been penetrated and air is being exchanged with the outside.

40: a. This condition is a tension pneumothorax.

41: a. Sealing the wound with an occlusive dressing is the appropriate treatment for a sucking chest wound.

42: b. In the paradoxical movement of a flail chest, the flail segment moves in the opposite direction from the rest of the chest cage.

43: b. Treatment for vaginal bleeding should not include the placement of any dressing within the vagina.

44: a. Application of direct pressure is the best means of controlling bleeding from the male genitalia.

45: d. All of these statements are true.

46: b. Application of cold packs is the appropriate treatment for a direct blow to the scrotum.

47: b. An impaled object should be left in place and stabilized.

48: d. All of these are appropriate treatment.

49: d. All of these are appropriate treatment.

Practical Applications

Consider how you would act, and why, in the following situations.

1. You arrive at the scene of a 2-car accident. The patient you are surveying is 18 years old, conscious, has pain in the abdomen. Pupils are equal, slightly dilated, and slow to react to light. Skin is cold and clammy. Pulse is rapid, weak, and regular. Blood pressure is low and declines with ensuing readings. The patient is thirsty and nauseous. There are no marks or bruises on the head.

2. Your patient was involved in an auto accident. Your survey indicates a possible right-lower rib fracture. Closer inspection reveals an open wound which makes sucking sounds each time the patient inhales and exhales. After you adequately stabilize the wound site with an occlusive dressing and immobilize the fractured ribs, you notice that the patient seems to be experiencing greater dyspnea. The pulse is weak; blood pressure is low; and the veins in the neck are bulging.

3. You find your patient in the street, unconscious and lying face down with a knife sticking into his back below the right scapula. Your primary survey finds a snoring sound on inspiration. The pulse is 100 and weak. Blood pressure is 110/80.

4. Your survey of the driver involved in a motor vehicle accident indicates no neck, back, or head injury. The patient is conscious and alert, but is experiencing chest pain when he inhales. His respirations are rapid and shallow. He is clutching the side of his chest and won't let go long enough for you to perform a survey.

5. You are called to a motor vehicle accident. The driver is found lying across the front seat. The patient is cyanotic. The steering wheel is bent out of shape. When you open his shirt there are no obvious lacerations, but his chest shows paradoxical motion.

6. A young man has been stabbed in the upper right chest with a knife. When you arrive, the knife has been removed. The patient is cyanotic, and breathing is difficult. The wound site was sucking air, and has been bandaged with an occlusive bandage by a first responder. While en route to the hospital, cyanosis deepens; pulse and blood pressure indicate increasing shock; and dyspnea also increases. You notice the trachea has moved from the midline toward the uninjured side.

7. A driver of a car involved in a motor vehicle accident is found behind a bent steering wheel. He is cyanotic and in respiratory distress. He has tenderness and pain along the right side of his chest. All chest movements appear normal. Vitals are: pulse, 130; respirations, 30, labored and shallow; blood pressure, 100/50.

8. A 23-year-old male complains of sudden shortness of breath associated with a sharp pain high on his left chest. He tells you he has no prior cardiac or respiratory history. Lung sounds are clear although slightly diminished on his left side. Pulse is 120; respirations are 26 and shallow; blood pressure is 100/70.

9. Your patient is the victim of a motor vehicle accident. She is found sitting behind the wheel wearing a seat belt. She is conscious and complains that her stomach hurts. She winces as you survey her pelvic girdle. There are no apparent marks or bruises to the head; the pupils are equal and reactive to light; all motor responses are good. BP is 100/70; respirations are 18; pulse is 120.

10. You are called to treat the victim of a knife fight. The victim is found doubled over and has several lacerations of the arms and hands. Breathing is rapid and shallow. His shirt is bloodied in the abdominal area. Visual survey shows an 8-inch loop of intestine protruding from the abdominal wall. His pulse is 100; blood pressure is 95/40.

11. A man working on a lathe in a home shop was struck in the abdomen by a wood chisel. You find him lying on his back, surrounded by a pool of blood. The chisel is still impaled in the abdomen. Respirations are 30 and shallow; pulse is 134; blood pressure is 80/40.

12. You respond to a home and find a 38-year-old woman lying in bed. She complains of tenderness in the right upper quadrant that restricts her movement because of the pain. She informs you that the condition has developed over the past few hours and that she generally gets severe indigestion after eating fatty foods. There is no other medical history. Vitals are: pulse, 90; respirations, rapid and shallow; blood pressure, 120/80.

13. You are called to a home where a young boy has caught his penis in the zipper of his pants. His mother tells you that she tried to unzip it but was unable to because of the pain it caused. There is slight bleeding around the zipper and the child is frightened. His vitals are normal except for an elevated pulse rate.

14. You respond to find a woman in her 20s with an object inserted in her vagina. She is bleeding profusely from the vaginal orifice. Vitals are: pulse, 130 and thready; respirations, 26 and rapid; blood pressure, 100/60.

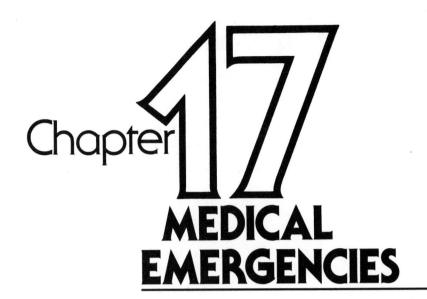

Chapter 17
MEDICAL EMERGENCIES

Comprehensive Questions

1. What is the cause of angina pectoris? What is its clinical picture?

2. What is a myocardial infarction? Describe its clinical picture.

3. Why is chest pain reduced by rest and/or nitroglycerin in angina pectoris but not in myocardial infarction?

4. What is congestive heart failure? Describe its clinical picture.

5. Explain the process by which congestive heart failure produces pulmonary edema, and describe the clinical picture.

6. Why is a patient with any suspected cardiac condition not permitted to walk? Why is he transported in a sitting position?

7. Describe the clinical picture of a patient suffering a CVA.

8. Describe the condition of the lungs of a patient with emphysema. How does this condition compromise the patient's respiration?

9. What is asthma? Compare the clinical picture of asthma with that of emphysema.

10. What is diabetes mellitus? Compare the clinical picture of diabetic coma with that of insulin shock.

11. Why is the administration of glucose an indicated treatment for any diabetic patient regardless of the cause of his condition?

Performance Skills

The treatment of medical emergencies requires the informed selection and specialized application of many of the skills acquired at earlier stages of the course. The primary new skill required is the ability to recognize the different medical conditions that may present themselves, and select the proper treatment. These conditions include the following:

angina pectoris
acute myocardial infarction
congestive heart failure
cerebrovascular accident
asthma
emphysema
hyperventilation syndrome
diabetic coma
insulin shock
fever
convulsions
unconsciousness of undetermined origin

Reference Data

All elements of the clinical picture of a condition will not always be present in every case.

1. **Clinical picture of angina pectoris**
   a. chest pain
      1) sub-sternal; may radiate to neck or jaw, left arm, or both arms
      2) squeezing or crushing in nature
      3) mild to moderate in intensity
      4) lasting no more than 15 minutes
      5) incited by exercise or stress
      6) alleviated by rest or nitroglycerine
   b. may be no associated symptoms though in some cases diaphoresis, shortness of breath, and nausea will be present

2. **Clinical picture of acute myocardial infarction**
   a. chest pain
      1) sub-sternal; may radiate to neck or jaw, left arm, or to both arms
      2) squeezing or crushing in nature
      3) severe in intensity
      4) usually lasting more than 30 minutes
      5) may occur without exercise or stress
      6) not alleviated by rest or nitroglycerine
   b. diaphoresis
   c. dyspnea
   c. nausea and vomiting
   e. weakness
   f. feeling of impending death

3. **Clinical picture of congestive heart failure**
   a. dyspnea with rapid, labored breathing
   b. elevated pulse
   c. rales or fluid sounds in the lungs
   d. pink, frothy sputum
   e. cyanosis in advanced cases
   f. if right heart failure ensues, neck veins may be distended

4. **Clinical picture of cerebrovascular accident**
   a. consciousness may be diminished
   b. difficulty with speech
   c. headache
   d. possible convulsions
   e. weakness or paralysis on one side of the body indicated by:
      1) unequal hand grasps
      2) loss of facial muscle tone

5. **Clinical picture of asthma**
   a. wheezing; with long, forced exhalations
   b. patient sitting up straight, often leaning forward
   c. chest hyperinflated
   d. patient may be cold and clammy

6. **Clinical picture of emphysema**
   a. dyspnea, with the use of neck and shoulder muscles to inhale
   b. pursing of lips to exhale
   c. rapid pulse
   d. patient commonly has a barrel-like chest, and is often thin

7. **Clinical picture of hyperventilation syndrome**
   a. carpopedal spasm
   b. dizziness
   c. tingling or numbness of hands and feet and around the mouth
   d. stabbing chest pains
   e. high rate of respiration
   f. elevated pulse
   g. possible fainting

8. **Clinical picture of diabetic coma**
   a. red, dry skin
   b. rapid, deep respirations
   c. weak, rapid pulse
   d. acetone or fruity breath odor
   e. lowered blood pressure
   f. varying degrees of consciousness

9. **Clinical picture of hypoglycemia**
   a. pale, moist, cold skin
   b. normal respirations
   c. full, rapid pulse
   d. weakness and headache
   e. irritable, nervous behavior
   f. seizures and coma in severe cases

Review Questions

Select the correct answer for each of the following questions. There is only *one* correct answer for each.

1. To "cool down" a child with a fever of 105°, sponge with:
    a. a mixture of ice and water.
    b. tepid or cool water.
    c. alcohol.
    d. cold packs.

2. A patient is convulsing when you arrive. You should:
    a. insert a bitestick, even if force is required.
    b. administer oxygen by mask.
    c. insert an oropharyngeal airway.
    d. protect him from hurting himself.

3. After an epileptic seizure the patient should be advised to:
    a. take aspirin.
    b. walk around.
    c. drink coffee.
    d. sleep or rest.

4. Convulsions may be caused by:
    a. high fever.
    b. epilepsy.
    c. brain injury.
    d. all of these.

5. Your survey of an unconscious woman determines that her pupils are of unequal size and her left side is paralyzed. You should transport her:
    a. on her back in the shock position.
    b. on her back with her head elevated.
    c. on her left side to face the aisle.
    d. on her right side with the cot in backwards.

6. Your patient is a 16-year-old who has just been involved in a family argument. Examination reveals rapid, deep ventilation, dizziness, numbness around the mouth, and tingling fingers. Suspect:
    a. an overdose of valium.
    b. asthma.
    c. hyperventilation syndrome.
    d. a convulsive disorder.

7. In cases of unconsciousness of unknown cause, the EMT should:
    a. place the patient in the coma position.
    b. monitor the patient's airway and respiration.
    c. give oxygen.
    d. all of the above.

8. Fluid sounds in the lungs without trauma may indicate:
    a. a diabetic emergency.
    b. shock.
    c. cerebrovascular accident.
    d. a cardiac emergency.

9. An elderly female patient is having difficulty breathing even while using 2 pillows to raise her head. When you depress the swollen-looking skin about the patient's ankles, the depression remains when you remove your finger. While transporting, you should:
    a. give oxygen and elevate the legs to treat for shock.
    b. put air splints on both legs to force blood to the heart.
    c. give oxygen and transport the patient in a sitting position.
    d. place her in the prone position.

10. A problem often associated with a heart attack patient is:
    a. getting the victim appropriately dressed.
    b. transporting the victim, as he often doesn't want to believe he is having an attack.
    c. getting automobiles to yield the right of way to your red lights and siren.
    d. convincing the emergency room staff you have a heart attack victim.

11. A 39-year-old man experienced chest pain to the left of his sternum immediately after playing touch football with his children. When you arrive he is shaken, but not in pain. What do you suspect?
    a. Myocardial infarction.
    b. Angina pectoris.
    c. Congestive heart failure.
    d. Spontaneous pneumothorax.

12. A 54-year-old female suddenly collapses at the theater. The pupils are dilated and there is no detectable pulse or respiration. A medi-alert bracelet on her arm states she is a diabetic. This patient is most likely suffering from:
    a. diabetic coma.
    b. insulin shock.
    c. cerebrovascular accident.
    d. cardiac arrest.

13. Many older people have a condition in which the pumping action of the heart is inadequate. This may cause a fluid accumulation in the body. What is the name of this condition?
    a. Angina pectoris.
    b. Myocardial infarction.
    c. Congestive heart failure.
    d. Cerebrovascular accident.

14. An EMT can assist a conscious patient to take a prescribed nitroglycerin pill by seeing that:
    a. he chews it thoroughly.
    b. he swallows it with a glass of water.
    c. he places it under his tongue.
    d. all of the above.

15. A patient suspected of suffering from angina should be treated as if he:
    a. suffered an MI.
    b. was a victim of a CVA.
    c. was having a diabetic emergency.
    d. was a low priority patient.

16. In caring for a patient with a suspected heart attack, the EMT should:
    a. allow him to walk only to the stretcher.
    b. allow him to move from his bed to the stretcher.
    c. not allow him to lift his own weight.
    d. assist and support him as he walks.

17. A 65-year-old male with a history of heart disease has a sudden onset of profuse sweating with fatigue. You should suspect:
    a. a cerebrovascular accident.
    b. myocardial infarction.
    c. angina pectoris.
    d. congestive heart failure.

18. A pulsating abdominal mass is suggestive of:
    a. adrenal insufficiency.
    b. appendicitis.
    c. aneurysm.
    d. pulmonary edema.

19. A patient having a heart attack experiences pain due to:
    a. anxiety.
    b. decreased oxygen supply to heart muscle.
    c. arrythmia.
    d. decreased nutrient supply to heart muscle.

20. Your patient is having sub-sternal pain, and you suspect he is experiencing a myocardial infarction. He tells you he has emphysema. In spite of that, you have been giving him oxygen at 4 liters per minute and he continues to by cyanotic. You should now:
    a. have him breathe into a paper bag.
    b. insert an airway and ventilate with positive pressure.
    c. increase the oxygen flow rate but be prepared to assist ventilation.
    d. reduce the oxygen flow.

21. The most serious result of heart attack is:
    a. paralysis.
    b. mental depression.
    c. severe pain in the chest.
    d. cardiac arrest.

22. The care and treatment of the patient with an acute abdomen includes:
    a. administering oxygen.
    b. being prepared for vomiting, and positioning the patient to guard against aspiration or choking.
    c. allowing the patient to flex his legs and lie in a comfortable position.
    d. all of the above.

23. A 52-year-old man is lying on the couch and is unable to sit up without help. He is having trouble explaining why you were called; his speech is slurred and incoherent. You find his hand grasps are unequal, and there is drooling. You should suspect he:
    a. is having an MI.
    b. has had a CVA.
    c. has muscular dystrophy.
    d. is intoxicated or under the influence of drugs.

24. Which of the following symptoms will the EMT see in many patients with cerebrovascular accidents?
    a. Unequal pupils.
    b. Paralysis of the lower extremities.
    c. Paralysis on one side of the body.
    d. Stiffness of the neck.

25. Symptoms of heart attack may:
    a. be mild and ignored, or attributed to some other cause.
    b. occur suddenly without warning.
    c. subside and return.
    d. all of the above.

26. Nitroglycerin is often prescribed for the treatment of:
    a. CVA.
    b. angina pectoris.
    c. myocardial infarction.
    d. congestive heart failure.

27. A major consideration with a heart attack patient is:
    a. to transport the patient to the hospital with as little delay as possible.
    b. not to give too high a concentration of oxygen.
    c. to force the patient to take oxygen by mask.
    d. transport the patient in a prone position.

28. The blocking of a coronary artery causes a condition known as:
    a. congestive heart failure.
    b. myocardial infarction.
    c. stroke.
    d. angina pectoris.

29. The condition resulting when the arteries become roughened and narrowed by fatty deposits that harden is:
    a. coronary embolism.
    b. arteriosclerosis.
    c. thrombosis.
    d. occlusion.

30. Nitroglycerin relieves cardiac pain by:
    a. deadening the sense of pain.
    b. decreasing cardiac output.
    c. dilating blood vessels.
    d. increasing blood pressure.

31. The condition that results when the blood supply to part of the brain is cut off, impairing the function of the cells in that part of the brain, is called:
    a. heart attack.
    b. cerebrovascular accident.
    c. chronic heart failure.
    d. angina pectoris.

32. Recent studies have shown that instant glucose is only effective when it is:
    a. swallowed.
    b. placed under the tongue.
    c. placed between the gum and cheek.
    d. chewed.

33. What effect does insulin have on blood sugar?
    a. Causes it to be produced.
    b. Causes it to be utilized.
    c. Causes it to enter the liver.
    d. Has no effect on blood sugar.

34. When transporting an unconscious patient, you should:
    a. rush him to the hospital.
    b. place him in a sitting position.
    c. position him on his side so that his airway can be managed.
    d. allow him to be as comfortable as possible.

35. Diabetic coma may be caused by:
    a. not taking insulin.
    b. not eating properly.
    c. an infection of any kind.
    d. all of the above.

36. When an EMT cannot determine whether a patient is stuporous because of insulin shock or because of diabetic coma, he should:
    a. administer glucose and protect the patient from aspiration.
    b. encourage the patient to take an insulin solution orally, if there is no danger that the patient will aspirate.
    c. encourage the patient to self-administer additional insulin.
    d. defer treatment and transport the patient to the hospital.

37. An excess of insulin—which may result when a diabetic patient has taken too much insulin, has not eaten, or has over-exercised—causes a condition known as:
    a. pancreatitis.
    b. diabetic coma.
    c. gluconeogenesis.
    d. insulin shock.

38. A 26-year-old male patient complains of intense thirst, headache, and vomiting. The skin is red and dry, blood pressure is low, and pulse is rapid. There is a sweet, fruity smell on his breath. This patient is probably suffering from:
    a. pancreatitis.
    b. diabetic ketoacidosis.
    c. insulin shock.
    d. gluconeogenesis.

39. Use all of the following for treatment of asthma *except*:
    a. sitting position.
    b. humidified oxygen.
    c. reassurance.
    d. insert an airway.

40. A patient with spontaneous pneumothorax is treated for a:
    a. very severe compression of the chest.
    b. rupture in the lung allowing air into the pleural space.
    c. condition in which air is leaking out of the lungs and collecting under the patient's skin.
    d. condition in which blood is present in the chest cavity.

41. When treating patients with emphysema, an EMT should *not*:
    a. explain the treatment sequence.
    b. transport the patient sitting up.
    c. help the patient to take his medication.
    d. administer large amounts of oxygen.

42. When treating a conscious asthma patient, you should:
    a. help him take any prescribed medication as often as necessary to provide relief.
    b. help him take any prescribed medication, being careful not to exceed prescribed dosage.
    c. prevent him from taking any medication.
    d. transport immediately.

43. In a certain medical disorder, spasm of the bronchial muscles constrict the bronchial tubes. The bronchi become congested, and normal breathing becomes progressively more difficult. This condition is known as:
    a. emphysema.
    b. asphyxia.
    c. asthma.
    d. pneumonia.

44. Which of the following is *not* a communicable disease?
    a. Chicken pox.
    b. Mumps.
    c. Measles.
    d. Emphysema.

45. Before transporting a patient with a suspected or known communicable disease, the crew should:
    a. remove all unnecessary equipment from the vehicle.
    b. carry a disposable mask and gown.
    c. use disposable equipment whenever possible.
    d. all of the above.

46. Which of the following should be done after transporting a patient with a known communicable disease?
    a. Ambulance personnel should be notified and possibly immunized by the emergency department.
    b. The ambulance should be checked and decontaminated.
    c. All linen and miscellaneous articles used on that call should be treated as contaminated.
    d. All of the above.

47. Which of the following is a method of transmitting communicable disease?
    a. Droplet infection, coughing.
    b. Indirect contact, handling contaminated objects.
    c. Direct contact, touching.
    d. All of the above.

Answers to Review Questions

1: b. Tepid or cool water should be used to sponge down a child with a fever; *never* use alcohol or ice water.

2: d. The EMT should protect the convulsing patient so he does not injure himself.

3: d. After an epileptic seizure, a patient is advised to rest or sleep.

4: d. All of these conditions can cause convulsions.

5: c. This patient should be transported on her left side to face the aisle.

6: c. A clinical picture of dizziness, numbness around the mouth, and tingling fingers indicates hyperventilation syndrome.

7: d. These are all steps in the proper care of an unconscious patient.

8: d. Of the choices given, only a cardiac emergency would cause fluid sounds in the lungs.

9: c. This patient has chronic congestive heart failure and should be given oxygen and transported in a sitting position.

10: b. Very often the victim of a cardiac emergency does not want to accept that this condition exists. The EMT must be professional and reassuring, but firm.

11: a. A first episode at age 39 is probably an acute coronary.

12: d. The absence of pulse and respiration in this patient indicates cardiac arrest.

13: c. Ineffective pumping of the heart which results in fluid buildup is called congestive heart failure.

14: c. A nitroglycerin tablet should be placed under the tongue and allowed to dissolve and be absorbed.

15: a. The EMT should treat the patient with angina as he would any victim of a myocardial infarction.

16: c. The patient suspected of having a heart attack should not be allowed to lift his own weight.

17: d. These symptoms and the patient's history indicate myocardial infarction.

18: c. A pulsating abdominal mass is indicative of an aneurysm.

19: b. The pain of a heart attack is due to a decrease in the supply of blood and oxygen to the heart muscle.

20: c. In this situation, the EMT has no choice but to increase the flow rate and be prepared should respiratory arrest occur. It is suggested that the patient be allowed to hold the mask.

21: d. The most serious result of a heart attack is cardiac arrest.

22: d. All of these are included in the proper treatment of a patient with an acute abdomen.

23: b. The EMT should suspect that this patient has had a CVA (cerebrovascular accident or stroke).

24: c. Paralysis of one side.

25: d. All are true of a heart attack.

26: b. Nitroglycerin, which acts to dilate the blood vessels and allow more oxygenated blood to reach the heart, is often prescribed for angina pectoris.

27: a. The EMT should make every effort to transport the patient to the hospital as quickly as possible.

28: b. A myocardial infarction is caused when the coronary arteries become blocked. Oxygenated blood cannot reach the heart muscle and tissue dies.

29: b. Arteriosclerosis is the condition caused by the hardening of fatty deposits in the arteries.

30: c. Nitroglycerin relieves cardiac pain by dilating blood vessels, thus allowing more oxygenated blood to reach the heart muscle.

31: b. A cerebrovascular accident results when the blood supply to part of the brain is cut off and cellular function is impaired.

32: a. Glucose is absorbed into the blood fastest when it is swallowed. It is not absorbed through the mucosa of the mouth.

33: b. Insulin causes blood sugar to be utilized.

34: c. An unconscious patient should be placed in coma position facing the aisle so that his airway can be managed.

35: d. Diabetic coma can be caused by any or all of these factors.

36: a. The EMT should administer glucose in either case and monitor the patient's airway.

37: d. Insulin shock (reaction) is caused by an excess of insulin due to any of the factors listed.

38: b. These symptoms indicate diabetic ketoacidosis.

39: d. An airway should not be used when treating an asthmatic patient.

40: b. Treat this patient for a rupture in the lung that allows air to leak into the pleural space.

41: d. Large amounts of oxygen (high liter flow) should not be administered to any patient suffering from a chronic obstructive lung disease.

42: b. The EMT should assist the asthma patient to take his medication, being careful not to exceed the prescribed dosage.

43: c. Asthma is caused by constriction of the bronchi and the accumulation of mucus.

44: d. All are communicable diseases except emphysema.

45: d. All of these precautions should be observed if the crew knows in advance that they will be transporting a patient with a communicable disease.

46: d. All of these should be done after transporting a patient with a communicable disease.

47: d. All are methods of transmitting communicable diseases.

Practical Applications

Consider how you would act, and why, in the following situations.

1. A 35-year-old man collapsed while jogging alone. When you arrive, he is incoherent with a bloody froth at his lips. Your survey indicates no trauma or fracture. A few minutes later his wife arrives and tells you that he hasn't had an epileptic seizure in over 9 years, hasn't taken any medication lately, and hasn't eaten since last night.

2. A 50-year-old man suddenly experienced pain in his chest and left arm while cutting his lawn. He came inside to lie down. He tells you that he took his last little white pill a few days ago and he just called the drugstore for more pills. The druggist immediately called the ambulance. The man is lying on a couch. His blood pressure is 90/70; respirations are labored; pulse is 130.

3. On a call to a nursery school you find a young child lying on the ground with his arms and legs in spasmodic contractions. His face is cyanotic and there is a slight frothing at the mouth.

4. Responding to a call you find an infant with a fever of 105°. Before transporting the infant to a medical facility you decide to begin emergency care.

5. You respond to a home late at night and find a 60-year-old female lying unconscious at the bottom of a stairway. She has an open fracture of the left forearm. A family member informs you that she went to bed early because she had a bad headache and that she must have gotten up for some reason. Blood pressure is 190/150; respirations are shallow; pulse is rapid and weak; pupils are unequal.

6. You are called to the home of a 48-year-old man who is lying on a couch. He is having trouble explaining why he called. His speech is slurred and he can't seem to find the right words to use. As you examine him, you find that his hand grasps are unequal and that his face seems to be "drooping" on one side. He is drooling slightly and is unable to sit up without help.

7. Your patient is a 48-year-old woman who has experienced a tightness in her chest for the last hour or two and is now having some nausea and difficulty breathing. Her only past illness was a hysterectomy 18 months ago. Her blood pressure is 124/86; respirations are 22; she seems concerned, but is relatively calm and controlled.

8. A 51-year-old fireman collapsed suddenly while performing his duties at a fire. The patient complains of severe chest pain radiating into the shoulder and down the left arm. The patient is diaphoretic and pale. There is no previous medical history. Respirations are 30 and shallow; pulse is 120; and blood pressure is 145/95.

9. You find a man whose car hit a tree head on. The man is nauseous and in severe pain. He complains of pain radiating down the left arm. The steering wheel is not buckled and the impact seems not to have been severe. He complains that he suffered a severe pain in the chest and lost control of his car. You smell no alcohol on his breath.

10. You find an unconscious male aged 40 on the floor next to his desk in an office. He is wearing a medi-alert bracelet that indicates he is diabetic. He is flushed and dry and has a fruity smell to his breath. Pulse is 80; respirations are rapid and deep; blood pressure is 130/70.

11. A 45-year-old man is found lying in an alleyway. He appears drowsy and confused. His speech is slurred and incoherent. His pulse is 90 and respirations are 28. His skin is very dry and his breath smells like nail polish remover. No other history is available.

12. You are called to a home where a young woman has been found unconscious at the bottom of a flight of stairs. She is lying on her back, apparently having fallen head first. She has a bruise over her left eye. Your survey indicates no apparent deformity but she is wearing a medi-alert bracelet that indicates "diabetic." Blood pressure is 130/90; respirations are 20 and shallow; pulse is 96.

13. You are called to an office to treat a 52-year-old man. When you arrive, he is found sitting at his desk, breathing heavily. He is red-faced, slightly overweight, and anxious. He tells you he summoned help because he suddenly felt that his heart was racing. His vitals are: pulse, 140 and bounding; respirations, 20 and deep; blood pressure, 220/130.

14. An elderly woman has called you to her home to treat her husband. You find him sitting in a chair in the bedroom next to an oxygen tank. His breathing is being assisted by a nasal cannula and he is dyspneic. His wife doesn't remember the name of his illness, but she says he has "breathing problems." Vitals are: pulse, 90; respirations, 36 and labored; blood pressure, 140/90.

15. You are called to a home to treat an 18-year-old female. She is breathing frantically at a very fast rate. She is lying on a couch and family members tell you that this condition developed suddenly after a family argument. Her pulse is 100; respirations are 60; and her blood pressure is 100/70.

16. You respond to a call for a youth having difficulty breathing. You find a 13-year-old girl sitting on a couch in a hot, dry room. Her respirations are labored. She appears frightened and her apprehension grows as she continues to have difficulty breathing. You hear a wheezing sound each time she exhales. The pulse is 120; respirations are 30; BP is 130/90.

17. An elderly gentlemen was referred to your care by the police because he was unable to walk unaided. His history indicates alcoholism. He repeats, "They're watching me," "They're chasing me." Vitals are normal.

18. An elderly man is seen at 2 A.M. at home. His wife tells you that he awoke and had great difficulty breathing. You note cyanosis around the lips, marked dyspnea, and gurgling sounds. His wife informs you that the doctor prescribed digitalis yesterday, but that otherwise his health has been OK. Vitals are: pulse, 140; respirations, 40; blood pressure, 150/100. Neck veins are distended.

19. You are called to treat a 65-year-old man who has developed respiratory difficulty. He complains of shortness of breath, and fluid sounds are heard when he breathes. He tells you that this attack isn't too bad—he's had attacks much worse. Your survey indicates his ankles appear to be "puffy." Pulse is 130; respiration is normal.

Chapter 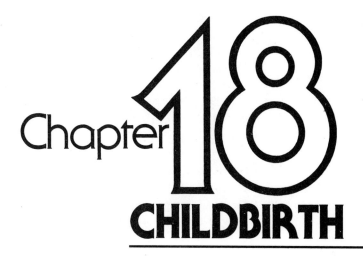 18
CHILDBIRTH

Comprehensive Questions

1. What are the factors the EMT must consider in determining whether a patient about to give birth should be transported or prepared for delivery at the scene?

2. Describe in sequence the steps in a normal field delivery.

3. Explain the function of the umbilical cord. Why is a prolapsed cord an emergency situation?

4. Describe the proper procedures when, in the course of a breech birth, the head does not deliver.

5. Describe the procedures to be followed when the presenting part in a delivery is an arm or leg.

6. Outline the care which should be given to the newborn upon delivery.

7. Describe the physiology of birth and the stages of labor.

Performance Skills

1. Determine the interval between contractions.

2. Assess a patient for, and recognize, crowning.

3. Assist a normal delivery.

4. Assist a delivery when the amniotic sac has not broken.

5. Assist a delivery when the presenting part is the buttocks or legs.

6. Clamp, tie, and cut the umbilical cord.

7. Control the mother's hemorrhage following the delivery of the placenta.

8. Assist and transport a mother with a prolapsed cord.

9. Assist in the delivery and transport of a premature baby.

Reference Data

1.

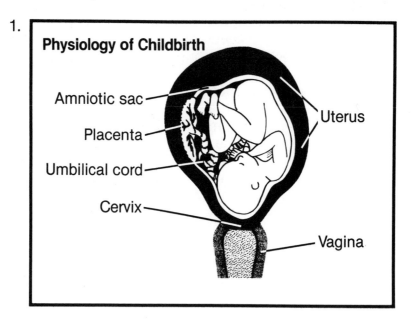

Physiology of Childbirth

Amniotic sac
Placenta
Umbilical cord
Cervix
Uterus
Vagina

2. **Transportation vs. delivery at the scene**
   In most areas, you should transport the expectant mother to the emergency department *if*:
   a. this is her first child *and*:
      1. contractions are 5 or more minutes apart.
      2. she does *not* have to strain or move her bowels.
   b. she has had a previous child *and*:
      1. contractions are 7 or more minutes apart.
      2. she does *not* have to strain or move her bowels.
   c. the previous children were delivered by Caesarean section.

   If these conditions are not met, examination for crowning will be the determining factor.

Review Questions

Select the correct answer for each of the following questions. There is only *one* correct answer for each.

1. A woman, pregnant for the first time, is having labor pains every 5 minutes. In this situation you should:
   a. prepare for imminent delivery.
   b. transport the woman to the hospital.
   c. hold the woman's legs together until the doctor arrives.
   d. tell the woman to relax between pains.

2. If difficulties arise during the delivery of the upper shoulder, the EMT can assist by:
   a. gently pulling at the baby's shoulders.
   b. gently guiding the baby's head downward.
   c. gently guiding the baby's head upward.
   d. gently pushing his gloved hand into the vagina.

3. Following delivery, the placenta should be saved and transported to the hospital because the:
   a. hospital staff can determine if the placenta has been completely expelled.
   b. shape of the placenta will suggest if there are any hidden deformities in the newborn.
   c. blood content of the placenta can be used if the newborn needs a transfusion.
   d. weight of the placenta is recorded for legal purposes.

4. In order to decide whether or not to transport an expectant mother to the hospital, the EMT should:
   a. ask the mother if she is having her first baby.
   b. ask her how long she has been in labor.
   c. ask her if she feels as though she has to move her bowels.
   d. all of the above.

5. You should suspect "multiple" delivery if:
   a. the mother's abdomen is unusually large before delivery.
   b. the mother's abdomen remains large after delivery.
   c. labor pains continue after one baby is delivered.
   d. all of the above.

6. If a woman is having her first baby, labor will usually last for approximately:
   a. 15 hours.
   b. 5 hours.
   c. 2 hours.
   d. 1 hour.

7. Following the normal delivery of a newborn, you notice that bleeding from the vagina is excessive. How should you attempt to reduce this bleeding?
    a. Compress the uterus toward the vagina.
    b. Pack sterile absorbant material into the vagina.
    c. Elevate the mother's feet and legs and massage the uterus.
    d. Elevate the mother's head and shoulder and rush her to the hospital.

8. When dealing with a prolapsed cord, the EMT should place the mother in an exaggerated shock position, and then:
    a. gently push the baby's head back into the vagina.
    b. rush her to the hospital; there is nothing he can do.
    c. discuss a course of action with a physician via radio or telephone.
    d. keep the cord moist and transport immediately.

9. If this is the expectant mother's first child, and the interval of contractions is short, you should:
    a. examine for crowning, then decide to transport or not.
    b. transport immediately.
    c. prepare to deliver at home.
    d. transport slowly, avoiding potholes.

10. Determine if this is the expectant mother's first child because:
    a. the data is needed by the hospital.
    b. labor will be longer with the first birth.
    c. labor will be shorter with the first birth.
    d. labor will be longer if there were other births.

11. If the amniotic sac does not break during delivery, the EMT should:
    a. do nothing; it will burst eventually.
    b. wait until after delivery and strip with sterile scissors.
    c. puncture it and remove it from around the baby's nose and mouth.
    d. transport immediately.

12. When the baby's head is delivered, the EMT should support the head by:
    a. maintaining finger pressure against the center of the baby's skull.
    b. placing the palm of his hand firmly against the baby's skull.
    c. distributing his fingers evenly around the baby's head.
    d. none of these.

13. If bleeding continues from the umbilical cord after clamping and cutting, the EMT should:
    a. clamp the cord again, close to the original closure.
    b. unclamp the cord and tie.
    c. apply a sterile pressure dressing.
    d. transport the baby immediately.

14. Following delivery of the baby's head, immediately:
    a. check the mother for bleeding.
    b. check the position of the umbilical cord.
    c. suction the nose and mouth.
    d. apply gentle pressure over the mother's abdomen.

15. The fetus develops within the:
    a. umbilicus.
    b. placenta.
    c. uterus.
    d. fundus.

16. While developing, the fetus is in a fluid-filled bag called the:
    a. uterine sac.
    b. placental sac.
    c. perineal sac.
    d. amniotic sac.

17. In a normal delivery the baby's face is initially turned:
    a. up.
    b. to the right.
    c. down.
    d. to the left.

18. During breech birth, the baby's head usually will delivery of its own accord. However, suffocation will occur if the head is not delivered within:
    a. 4 minutes.
    b. 3 minutes.
    c. 2 minutes.
    d. 1 minute.

19. The growing fetus receives its nourishment from the mother through the:
    a. amniotic fluid.
    b. vagina.
    c. placenta.
    d. uterus.

20. In preparing the patient for delivery, the EMT should:
    a. place the patient on a bed with a sheet under her buttocks.
    b. provide a bucket in case of vomiting.
    c. position a second EMT, or perhaps the father, at the mother's head.
    d. all of the above.

21. The danger of a prolapsed umbilical cord is that:
    a. the baby may suffocate due to lack of oxygen.
    b. the cord may strangle the baby.
    c. the cord may pull the placenta free when the baby delivers.
    d. all of the above.

22. An arm or leg presentation is an indication that the baby has shifted into such a position that:
     a. 2 EMTs are required to handle the delivery.
     b. normal delivery is not possible and special obstetrical procedures must be employed.
     c. the EMT must place his hands in the mother's vagina and position the baby for delivery.
     d. none of the above.

23. A baby weighing less than 5½ pounds at birth:
     a. is by definition an immature baby.
     b. is by definition a premature baby.
     c. is one that is born before the sixth month of pregnancy.
     d. is one that is born before the third month of pregnancy.

24. The following steps should be taken to care for a premature baby:
     a. keep warm by wrapping in a blanket and then in aluminum foil.
     b. clear mouth and nose of fluid and mucus.
     c. prevent bleeding from the cord.
     d. all of the above.

Answers to Review Questions

1: b. In most areas the EMT will have sufficient time to transport the patient to the emergency department if the contractions are 5 minutes apart.

2: b. The EMT can assist the delivery of the upper shoulder by gently guiding the baby's head downward.

3: a. The hospital staff can determine if the placenta has been completely expelled, reducing the danger of infection in the mother.

4: d. The EMT should determine the answers to all of these questions, and examine the patient for crowning, to determine if there is time to transport her.

5: d. All of these are indicators of multiple delivery.

6: a. Labor with a first child usually lasts about 15 hours.

7: c. The EMT should elevate the mother's feet and legs and gently massage the uterus to control vaginal bleeding.

8: c. Since obstetricians differ on what is considered the preferred treatment, the EMT should discuss a course of action with the patient's obstetrician or the emergency department physician and follow his instructions.

9: a. The EMT should use the examination for crowning as the criterion for whether or not to transport.

10: b. Labor will be longer with the first child.

11: c. If the sac has not broken, the EMT should puncture it and remove it from around the baby's nose and mouth.

12: c. The EMT should distribute his fingers evenly around the baby's head to avoid putting pressure on the "soft spots" of the skull.

13: a. The cord should be clamped or tied again, close to the original clamps. The first clamps should not be removed.

14: b. The EMT should check the position of the umbilical cord to determine that it is not pinched or has not become wrapped around the baby's neck.

15: c. The fetus develops within the mother's uterus.

16: d. The developing fetus is protected by the amniotic sac.

17: c. The baby's face initially is turned down, then rotates toward a thigh.

18: b. The infant may suffocate during a breech birth if the head is not delivered within 3 minutes.

19: c. The developing fetus receives its nourishment through the placenta.

20: d. All of these should be done when preparing to assist in a delivery at home.

21: a. The danger of a prolapsed cord is that it may become pinched, causing the baby to suffocate.

22: b. An arm or leg presentation is undeliverable without surgical assistance.

23: b. A premature baby is defined as one weighing less than 5½ pounds or one born before 8 months of pregnancy.

24: d. All of these are included in the proper care of a premature baby.

Practical Applications

Consider what you would do, and why, in the following situations.

1. You respond to a home to find a woman who is 8 months pregnant. She reports that her "water just broke and contractions are coming every 2 to 3 minutes." This will be her third child. Previous births were routine.

2. You respond to a woman "having contractions" who states that she is 2 weeks overdue. This will be her first child. Her water has not broken, and contractions are 10 minutes apart.

3. You are called to assist a woman in labor who reports that she is full term. You assist in a normal birth. After suctioning the very small infant, you clamp and cut the cord. You notice that the mother's abdomen is still large. The placenta still has not delivered and contractions begin again 15 minutes later.

4. You respond to assist a woman who is reported to be full term and in labor. A visual inspection shows evidence of crowning. You prepare to assist in the birth. As the head delivers, you see that it is still enclosed by the amniotic sac.

5. You respond to a call for "a woman hemorrhaging." Your patient is a 26-year-old female with heavy vaginal bleeding. She recently (3 weeks ago) gave birth to her third child and appears very anxious. Her pulse is 120; respirations are 28; and blood pressure is 100/60.

6. Your patient is a woman who is in her fifth month of pregnancy. She is seated on the toilet holding a towel between her legs. She says she felt a need to move her bowels, and while "straining" her water broke and the fetus partially delivered. Upon inspection you see a fetus one-half delivered.

7. You are called to assist a woman who is full term. Her contractions are 2 minutes apart. You decide to deliver at the house. With the next contraction, the feet deliver.

8. A woman is experiencing severe labor pains. Her pains are 1½ minutes apart, and this will be her fourth child. Upon examination, you see the baby's head protruding from the vagina.

9. You assist in a normal birth. After suctioning the newborn, you clamp and cut the cord. Twenty minutes later the placenta still has not delivered.

10. Upon arriving at the scene, you see that a 6 inch loop of umbilical cord is protruding from the vagina. The mother tells you her water has broken. You feel no pulsation in the cord.

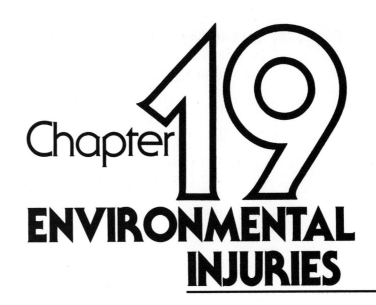

Chapter 19
ENVIRONMENTAL INJURIES

Comprehensive Questions

1. Describe the physiological make-up of the skin.

2. Describe the various degrees of burns, their appearance, and severity.

3. Why is the information gained by applying the "Rule of Nines" important in assessing a burn victim?

4. Discuss the systemic complications that can result from severe burns.

5. How does the inspiration of carbon monoxide affect the oxygenation of the blood?

6. Describe how the body reacts as it is exposed to colder and colder temperatures.

7. Describe what takes place in the airways and lungs in the course of a near drowning.

8. Explain why every near drowning victim must be taken to the emergency department, even if they have regained adequate spontaneous ventilation and full consciousness.

9. Explain how the body's reaction to immersion in cold water works to protect a victim of cold water near drowning.

10. Discuss the differences between heat exhaustion and heat stroke. Compare the clinical pictures of each.

Performance Skills

The proper treatment of environmental injuries requires the informed selection and specialized application of many manipulative skills acquired at earlier stages of the course.

The primary new skill introduced here is the ability to recognize the various conditions that might present themselves and to select the proper treatment for them. Previously learned skills in bandaging, oxygen administration, artificial ventilation, CPR, and other areas will be needed in this treatment. The conditions presented in this chapter include:

first, second, and third degree thermal burns
chemical burns
burns to the eye caused by light and chemicals
exposure to radiation
exposure to electrical shock
heat exhaustion
heat stroke
near drowning
cold water near drowning
hypothermia
frostbite
carbon monoxide poisoning

Reference Data

1.

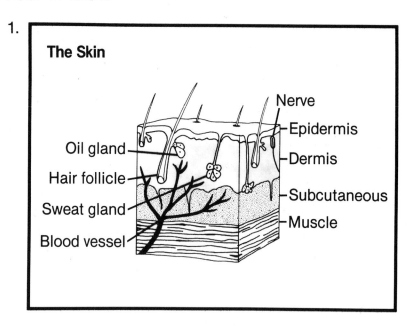

The Skin

Nerve
Epidermis
Oil gland
Dermis
Hair follicle
Sweat gland
Subcutaneous
Blood vessel
Muscle

2. **Types of burns**
   a. first degree burns: affect epidermis only; red, painful skin
   b. second degree burns: affect epidermis and part of dermis; blistering of skin
   c. third degree burns: affect epidermis and all of dermis; skin is white or charred

3.

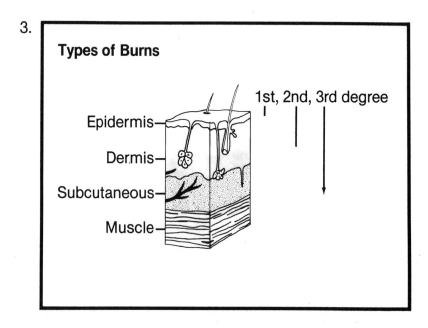

Types of Burns

1st, 2nd, 3rd degree
Epidermis
Dermis
Subcutaneous
Muscle

4.

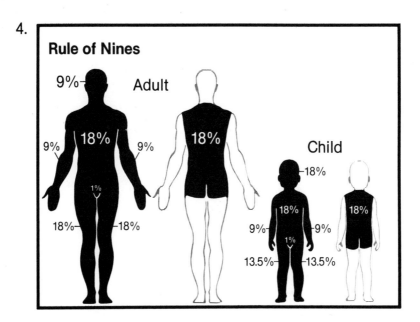

Rule of Nines

9% Adult

9% 18% 9%

18% 18%

1%

18% 18%

Child

18%

18% 18%

9% 9%

1%

13.5% 13.5%

5. **A burn is considered "severe" if:**
   a. the respiratory tract is involved
   b. first degree burns affect 75 percent or more of the body
   c. second degree burns affect 30 percent or more of the body
   d. third degree burns affect 10 percent or more of the body
   e. the affected areas include the face, hands, or feet
   f. the victim is a child, aged, or in poor health

6. **Clinical picture of heat exhaustion**
   a. pale, cold, clammy skin
   b. body temperature normal or below
   c. weakness, dizziness, or fainting; nausea
   d. vitals normal

7. **Stages of body cooling**
   a. shivering
   b. drowsiness—listlessness, muscular rigidity replaces shivering; thinking becomes unclear
   c. stupor, then unconsciousness; pulse and respiration slow
   d. extremities begin to freeze
   e. cardiac and respiratory centers of brain fail; cardiac arrhythmia, pulmonary edema
   f. death

8. **Clinical picture of heat stroke**
   a. warm, dry, flushed skin
   b. body temperature 105°F or above
   c. patient is disoriented or confused, eventually comatose
   d. pulse is initially rapid and full, but deteriorates to rapid and weak

9. **Cold water near drowning**
   a. mammalian diving reflex—Shunts blood from the rest of the body to the heart, lungs, and brain; is activated when the face is immersed in cold water
   b. immersion hypothermia—cold causes body metabolism to slow down and the need for oxygen to be reduced
   c. water temperature must be 68°F or below for this mechanism to function
   d. survival is a factor of water temperature, patient's age, weight, and length of immersion

Review Questions

Select the correct answer for each of the following questions. There is only *one* correct answer for each.

1. Carbon monoxide:
   a. paralyzes the respiratory muscles.
   b. destroys white cells.
   c. combines with hemoglobin more rapidly than oxygen.
   d. prevents blood from clotting.

2. A victim of hypothermia must be treated for shock because:
   a. as the body rewarms, blood vessels dilate.
   b. his rectal temperature may be below 81°F.
   c. his extremities are frozen.
   d. treating for shock is not required for hypothermia.

3. Gamma rays are the most dangerous type of ionizing radiation because they:
   a. can penetrate all but the densest materials.
   b. can damage body cells.
   c. do not have to be swallowed or inhaled.
   d. all of the above.

4. Alpha and beta particles are dangerous only if they are:
   a. swallowed along with food or drink.
   b. inhaled along with smoke or air.
   c. rubbed into a wound or onto the skin directly.
   d. all of these.

5. When treating patients involved in an accident with ionizing radiation, the EMT must be concerned about:
   a. the length of time he may be exposed.
   b. his distance from the radiation source.
   c. the amount of shielding between himself and the radiation source.
   d. all of these.

6. Applying a firm sterile dressing to a burn will benefit a victim in at least 3 ways. Which of the following is *not* one of these benefits?
   a. Prevents anemia.
   b. Reduces the probability of shock.
   c. Relieves pain.
   d. Prevents additional contamination.

7. The "Rule of Nines" is modified for an infant because:
   a. more area is taken up by the head and less by the legs.
   b. he is smaller than an adult.
   c. he has less skin to be affected.
   d. infants get severely burned.

8. Damage to a patient's skin may result in:
    a. loss of ability to fight infection.
    b. loss of ability to receive stimuli.
    c. loss of ability to control body temperature.
    d. all of the above.

9. "Shivering" indicates that the:
    a. body is trying to generate heat.
    b. body is losing its muscle control.
    c. circulatory system is straining.
    d. muscular system is straining.

10. The major purpose of emergency treatment for heat stroke is to:
    a. restore normal respiration.
    b. rid the body of extra heat.
    c. prevent convulsions.
    d. replace the salt lost through perspiration.

11. External heat must be provided to a hypothermia patient because:
    a. of the windchill factor
    b. his clothes are cold.
    c. his blood sugar is low.
    d. The body has lost its ability to generate heat.

12. Proper emergency medical treatment for burns of the eyes caused by light includes:
    a. covering both eyes with paper cones or cups.
    b. covering both eyes with sterile moist dressings.
    c. flushing both eyes with water or saline.
    d. transporting as a true emergency.

13. The accepted emergency medical treatment for both air embolism and "the bends" is:
    a. administer salt and water by mouth.
    b. recompression in a pressure chamber.
    c. apply hot packs and transport.
    d. have the patient move around to maintain circulation.

14. Alpha and beta particles are the least dangerous type of ionizing radiation because they:
    a. can be absorbed by clothing.
    b. have electrical charges.
    c. can penetrate all but the densest materials.
    d. all of the above.

15. A result of severe hypothermia is:
    a. cardiac thrombosis.
    b. cardiac arrhythmia.
    c. CVA.
    d. congestive heart failure.

16. The amount of damage ionizing radiation can do to a patient depends upon all of the following *except*:
    a. area of the body affected.
    b. distance from the radiation source.
    c. amount of shielding from the radiation source.
    d. age of the patient.

17. The amount of damage ionizing radiation can do to a patient depends upon all of the following *except*:
    a. strength of the radiation source.
    b. type of radiation.
    c. body size of the patient.
    d. duration of exposure to the radiation.

18. The least dangerous type of ionizing radiation is:
    a. alpha particles.
    b. beta particles.
    c. gamma rays.
    d. there is no least dangerous type.

19. After the apparent recovery of any near drowning victim, you should:
    a. insist on transporting the patient to an emergency department.
    b. advise him to see his doctor.
    c. allow him to go home.
    d. absolve yourself of legal responsibility.

20. A patient has had a long exposure to a very hot environment. When you arrive he is weak, dizzy, has a headache, and displays signs of shock.
    a. He has heat exhaustion. Move him to a cool area, treat for shock, and transport.
    b. He has heat stroke. Immediately cool the body with wet, cold towels or cold packs as you transport him.
    c. He has heat cramps. Move him to a cool area and let him sip salt water.
    d. None of the above.

21. A patient has been exposed to a very hot and humid climate for a long period of time. His skin is very hot, dry, and slightly reddish. His armpits are dry and his body temperature is 104°F. He reports that he feels ill but was not in the sun long.
    a. He has heat exhaustion. Move him to a cool area, treat for shock, and transport.
    b. He has heat stroke. Immediately cool the body with cold packs and transport.
    c. He has heat cramps. Move him to a cool area and have him sip salt water.
    d. None of the above.

22. Which of the following is *not* an indicator of heat stroke?
    a. Full and fast pulse.
    b. Moist skin.
    c. Nausea.
    d. High body temperature.

23. The major objective of emergency medical treatment for cases of exposure to heat is to:
    a. reduce the patient's body temperature to below 100°F if possible.
    b. have the patient sip as much salt water as possible.
    c. make the patient comfortable.
    d. transport the patient as rapidly as traffic allows.

24. After rewarming a frostbitten extremity, you can stimulate the return of circulation by:
    a. rhythmically raising and lowering the part.
    b. briskly massaging the affected part.
    c. increasing the temperature of the water.
    d. rubbing the part with snow.

25. A patient has frostbite. You are in a warm house, but are an hour or more from a medical facility due to bad weather. The proper emergency medical treatment includes:
    a. having the patient rub the affected area with his warm hand.
    b. rubbing the affected area with snow.
    c. placing the affected area in water of about 100°F.
    d. placing the affected area in ice water.

26. Hypothermia is:
    a. general cooling of the body.
    b. general heating of the body.
    c. superficial frostbite.
    d. trench foot.

27. For cases in which a patient has been exposed to cold and windy temperatures for a long period of time, you should:
    a. remove any cold, damp, or wet clothes.
    b. apply external heat carefully.
    c. place the patient in a blanket or sleeping bag to conserve body heat if no other sources of heat are available.
    d. all of the above.

28. Which of the following conditions occurs when the body's heat generation is lost?
    a. Frostbite.
    b. Trench foot.
    c. Chilblains.
    d. Hypothermia.

29. A general rule to follow when treating patients with frostbite is:
    a. a patient may not walk on a frozen limb.
    b. after thawing, the patient is a litter case.
    c. briskly massage the affected part to regain circulation.
    d. place a tourniquet between the frozen part and the heart.

30. When called to a suspected carbon monoxide poisoning, the EMT must be careful to:
    a. avoid being overcome himself.
    b. have enough oxygen in the ambulance.
    c. protect the patient's airway if he vomits.
    d. all of the above.

31. Carbon monoxide is a poison that is:
    a. inhaled.
    b. ingested.
    c. absorbed through the skin.
    d. injected into a vein.

32. An electric shock can cause cardiac arrest because it may:
    a. affect the electrical conduction of the heart.
    b. cause the heart to contract.
    c. cause blood vessels to dilate.
    d. cause blood vessels to constrict.

33. After assuring your safety, the initial act in approaching the victim of electrical shock is to:
    a. move the patient to a flat surface.
    b. check for the presence of respiration and a pulse.
    c. survey for injuries.
    d. administer a painful stimulus.

34. When a chemical splashes into an eye, the EMT should:
    a. neutralize the chemical, then flush out with water.
    b. irrigate the eye with water.
    c. simply cover the eye and rush to the hospital.
    d. rinse the eye with a commercial eyewash solution.

35. Alkali burns are more serious than acid burns because:
    a. alkali cannot be washed off.
    b. alkali causes "flash" burns.
    c. alkali penetrates deeper and acts longer.
    d. all of the above.

36. A 10-year-old boy was playing with matches and set his clothes on fire. You see blistering and leathery, charred areas. He has:
    a. second degree burns.
    b. third degree burns.
    c. mixed first and second degree burns.
    d. mixed second and third degree burns.

37. A third degree burn is:
    a. a burn that results in some blistering and a deep reddening of the skin.
    b. a full-thickness burn of the skin.
    c. limited to the most superficial layer of the epidermis and is characterized by a reddening of the skin.
    d. the least serious type of burn.

38. The "Rule of Nines" is used to:
    a. estimate degree of burn.
    b. estimate amount of surface affected.
    c. describe section of body involved.
    d. describe patient's condition.

39. The subcutaneous layer of the skin functions as:
    a. an insulator of the body.
    b. a waterproof layer.
    c. a container for pigment cells.
    d. a barrier against bacteria.

40. Sweat and oil glands are located in which layer of the skin?
    a. Epidermis.
    b. Dermis.
    c. Sebaceous.
    d. Subcutaneous.

41. Mouth-to-mouth or mouth-to-nose ventilation for a suspected drowning victim should be started:
    a. as soon as the patient is in the ambulance.
    b. as soon as the patient can be placed on a firm surface.
    c. in the water, if possible.
    d. when at least 2 EMTs are at the scene.

42. When called to treat a burn victim, which should you do first?
    a. Determine if the patient has spontaneous respiration and circulation.
    b. Apply moist sterile dressings.
    c. Apply cold packs.
    d. Make certain additional help is on the way.

43. In severe burn cases, shock usually results from:
    a. pain.
    b. emotional distress.
    c. anxiety about disfigurement.
    d. fluid loss.

44. Emergency treatment for thermal burns of the eyes includes:
    a. covering both eyes with sterile, dry dressings.
    b. covering both eyes with sterile, moist dressings.
    c. flushing both eyes with water or saline.
    d. simply transporting.

45. Factors that are key to the EMT in evaluating the seriousness of thermal burns include:
    a. degree of burn and section of body involved.
    b. degree of burn, section of body involved, percentage of body surface affected, and age of the patient.
    c. degree of burn, age of patient, size of patient.
    d. weight, height, age, and size of patient.

46. When the skin has been burned by unknown alkalis or acids, you should:
    a. after flushing for 20 minutes, neutralize with a mild solution of the opposite Ph.
    b. before flushing for 20 minutes, neutralize with a mild solution of the opposite Ph.
    c. do not neutralize, just flush with water for 20 minutes.
    d. transport immediately.

47. When a poison is inhaled, it has entered the body through the:
    a. respiratory tract.
    b. skin.
    c. body tissues.
    d. bloodstream.

48. Even if a human or animal bite involves no more than a small puncture or laceration, the EMT should:
    a. wash the wound with an antiseptic soap, if possible, or at least rinse it with running water.
    b. apply a constricting band on the heart side of the wound.
    c. apply a constricting band above and below the wound.
    d. liberally coat the wound with either mercurochrome or merthiolate.

49. First degree and minor second degree burns can be made less painful by:
    a. covering with a sterile burn pad.
    b. covering with a waterless type of ointment.
    c. spraying with burn ointment.
    d. applying cold towels.

50. A first degree burn is characterized by:
    a. deep reddening and blistering.
    b. reddening.
    c. charring.
    d. reddening, blistering, and charring.

51. The body's reaction in a cold water near drowning is significantly affected by:
    a. the patient's age.
    b. the water temperature.
    c. the time of immersion.
    d. all of the above.

52. In a case of cold water near drowning, immersion hypothermia causes:
    a. blood to be concentrated in the peripheral areas.
    b. the heart rate to increase and respirations to deepen.
    c. body metabolism to slow and oxygen need to decrease.
    d. all of the above.

53. The mammalian diving reflex is triggered when:
    a. body temperature falls below 90 degrees.
    b. the face is immersed in cold water.
    c. the body is immersed below 6 feet of water.
    d. all of the above.

Answers to Review Questions

1: c. Carbon monoxide combines with the hemoglobin of the red blood cells about 200 times faster than oxygen does.

2: a. The hypothermia patient must be treated for shock since relative hypovolemia can occur as the rewarmed blood vessels dilate.

3: d. All of these are characteristics of gamma rays.

4: d. All of these are conditions under which alpha and beta particles can be dangerous.

5: d. The EMT must be concerned with all of these when treating the victim of a radiation accident.

6: a. Applying a firm sterile dressing will not prevent anemia.

7: a. The "Rule of Nines" is modified for an infant because more area is taken up by its head and less by its legs as compared to an adult.

8: d. All of these can result when a patient's skin is damaged.

9: a. "Shivering" indicates that the body is trying to generate heat.

10: b. The major treatment for heat stroke is to rid the body of excess heat to prevent damage to the cells of the central nervous system.

11: d. Heat must be provided to a hypothermia patient because the body has exhausted its ability to generate heat.

12: b. The EMT should cover both eyes of the victim of light burns with moist sterile dressings.

13: b. Recompression in a pressure chamber is the proper emergency treatment for both air embolism and "the bends."

14: a. Alpha and beta particles can be absorbed by clothing.

15: b. Cardiac arrhythmia may result from severe hypothermia.

16: d. The age of the patient is not a factor in determining the damage done by ionizing radiation.

17: c. The body size of the patient is not a factor in determining the damage done by ionizing radiation.

18: a. Alpha particles are considered to be the least dangerous type of ionizing radiation.

19: a. All near-drowning victims should be examined and evaluated by an emergency department physician.

20: a. Move him to a cool area, treat for shock, and transport.

21: b. The patient is suffering from heat stroke. The EMT should immediately begin to cool his body and transport.

22: b. Moist skin is not an indicator of heat stroke. Dry skin is an indicator.

23: a. In all cases of exposure to heat, the patient's body temperature should be lowered to below 100°F, if possible.

24: a. After rewarming, circulation can be stimulated by raising and lowering the part. *Never* massage the part or rub it with snow.

25: c. A frostbitten part can be rewarmed in water at about 100°F. Use a thermometer to monitor the water temperature and add hot water as necessary.

26: a. Hypothermia is a general cooling of the body.

27: d. All of these are appropriate steps in the treatment of a patient that has had a prolonged exposure to cold.

28: d. Hypothermia occurs when the body's heat generating mechanism no longer functions.

29: b. While a patient can walk on a frostbitten leg, after rewarming, this patient must be transported on a cot to avoid additional tissue damage.

30: d. All of the above.

31: a. Carbon monoxide is inhaled and combines with the hemoglobin of the blood cells.

32: a. An electrical shock can affect the electrical conduction of the heart.

33: b. The EMT should determine that there is adequate respiration and circulation.

34: b. A chemical burn to the eyes should be irrigated with copious amounts of water.

35: c. An alkali penetrates deeper and acts longer than an acid.

36: d. This patient has mixed second and third degree burns. This is indicated by blisters (second degree) and charring (third degree).

37: b. A third degree burn is a full thickness burn and is of great seriousness.

38: b. The "Rule of Nines" is used to estimate the amount (percentage) of the body surface affected.

39: a. The subcutaneous layer of skin acts as an insulator.

40: b. Sweat and oil glands are located in the second layer—the dermis—of the skin.

41: c. Artificial ventilation should be started in the water, if possible.

42: a. The EMT should always conduct a primary survey before beginning a course of treatment.

43: d. A burn victim can go into shock due to fluid loss.

44: b. The EMT should cover both the patient's eyes with sterile, moist dressings, and transport.

45: b. The degree of the burn, the section of the body involved, the percentage of body surface affected, and the age of the patient should be considered when evaluating a burn.

46: c. The EMT should not waste time neutralizing the agent. Flushing with water for 20 minutes is more effective.

47: a. A poison is inhaled through the respiratory tract.

48: a. An animal or human bite should be washed with an antiseptic soap or flushed with running water.

49: d. Application of cold compresses will relieve the pain of first or second degree burns.

50: b. A first degree burn is characterized by reddening.

51: d. All of these factors affect the body's reaction in a cold water near drowning.

52: c. Immersion hypothermia causes the body metabolism to slow, decreasing the amount of oxygen needed.

53: b. The mammalian diving reflex is brought into effect when the face is immersed in cold water.

Practical Applications

Consider how you would act, and why, in the following situations.

1. A child has been bitten by a dog. There are several puncture marks and scratches on the child's lower legs. No other injuries are evident.

2. You are returning to headquarters from the hospital when the dispatcher advises you that the patient you just delivered is suspected of having meningitis.

3. You are called to a local marina to treat a swimmer who has been brought ashore by boat. The patient is a 28-year-old male who complains of painful joints. His recent history reveals onset of pain and headache 4 hours after scuba diving. Vitals show only slight elevation which you attribute to anxiety.

4. You respond to a local swimming pool. A young child was pulled from the water after a near drowning. When you arrive, the child is huddled under a large towel and is being held and comforted by his mother. The child is shivering and is very scared.

5. You are called to treat a victim of a scuba diving accident. When you arrive, others tell you that the victim surfaced suddenly and was unconscious. His skin appears blotchy and he has frothy blood about his nose and mouth. Vitals are: pulse, 140 and thready; respirations, 36 and shallow; blood pressure, 110/60.

6. The temperature is 25°F with a wind of 15 miles per hour. A middle-aged male is found beneath a park bench. He is semi-responsive and you smell alcohol about his body. His hands and feet are cold, pale, and solid. There is no evidence of injury.

7. A young hiker is found lying in the woods after being lost for 2 days. The weather has been windy and wet. Temperatures have ranged from 30°F to 40°F. The patient is unconscious with a pulse of 36 and a respiration rate of 8. No blood pressure is measurable and there are no signs of injury.

8. A young girl has fallen through the ice while skating. Other skaters have used ladders and ropes to remove her from the water. When you arrive, she is shivering under a blanket in front of a campfire. She complains of no other injury or problem.

9. A bakery worker complains of painful cramps in the arms and legs. He is diaphoretic and has a pulse of 120. Respirations are 24; blood pressure is 120/70. You find him trying to "walk off" the cramps. He complains of being very thirsty.

10. A young woman suddenly became ill during a tennis game on a hot day. She tells you that she became weak, dizzy, and nauseous. She appears ashen gray and her skin is cool and clammy. Her vitals are BP 100/60; pulse 118; respiration 20.

11. You respond to a roadside on a hot day where you find an unconscious male approximately age 40. Members of the road crew report that he has been working for 5 hours. There is no apparent mechanism of injury. His skin feels hot and dry; pulse is 124 and weak; respirations are 24 and shallow; blood pressure is 90/50.

12. You are called to a highway accident to treat a fireman who was exposed to an unknown radiation source while hosing down the accident site involving a truck carrying nuclear wastes. Vitals are normal. He complains of no injuries or sickness.

13. You are called to the local high school chemical lab. When you arrive, you find a student being held under a safety shower by the instructor. You learn that a chemistry setup exploded, splashing a mixture of chemicals on the student. All of his clothes and lab safety equipment are still on as he stands under the safety shower.

14. A worker in an industrial plant has spilled an unknown liquid all over the front of his work clothes. He complains of a burning sensation. His eyes are tearing and his sight is blurred, though his hair is dry.

15. You are called to the chemistry laboratory at the local high school. A 17-year-old boy has spilled a white powdered substance on his bare arm. He reports a severe burning pain on his arm, is anxious, and has no other apparent injuries.

16. A young man was filling his car battery with water and overfilled two of the cells. He tells you he used a plastic straw to "suck up" or siphon the excess and that some of the fluid got into his mouth. He now complains of a severe burning sensation in his mouth. He clears his throat and spits often as you question him.

17. A cement worker was carrying a sack of dry lime when suddenly it broke. His bare arms are covered with white powder when you arrive.

18. Your patient is a 40-year-old woman who burned her hand and lower arm while cooking with a gas stove. Her hand and arm appear reddish and there are several blisters on the back of her hand. She is seated at a kitchen table complaining of pain. Pulse is 90; respirations are 20; blood pressure is 140/90.

19. You are called to a house fire. When you arrive, firemen are carrying a victim from the house toward you. You see charred areas all along the backside of the victim's clothing. The patient has also suffered smoke inhalation and is coughing violently. A close inspection of the charred areas shows pale, dry, charred skin with fabric adhering to the edges of the burn.

20. You are called to a home on a hot summer day. Your patient is an 18-year-old girl who was at the beach all day. She is lying face down in bed, unable to move because of severe pain. Her back and legs are bright red. Pulse is 110; respirations are 18; blood pressure is 120/70.

21. An unconscious patient has been pulled from the burning wreckage of a car by a passerby. She has burns of the legs and chest. Respirations are 26 and irregular; pulse is 130 and weak; BP is 90/60.

22. A young woman received a searing burn to the face while cooking. When you arrive she is found sitting on the floor holding her face, screaming in pain. She rubs her eyes and complains that she can't see. Your survey finds "raw-looking" tissues around her eyelids. Pulse is 130; respirations are 40; blood pressure is 150/90.

23. Upon arriving at a home you find two distraught parents trying to undress a screaming youngster. They tell you that the child pulled a pan of hot grease off from the stove onto himself. He appears to have spilled grease from his shoulders to his feet.

24. A 26-year-old male is found at a construction site complaining of very painful eyes. He says he was welding for about 2 hours earlier that day and suddenly his eyes began to hurt. He says the pain lessens but does not go away when he closes his eyes. His pulse is 90; respirations are 20; blood pressure is 120/70.

25. You respond to an industrial accident where an electrician came in contact with live wires. The patient is a 53-year-old male with what appears to be a third degree burn across his palm. You find the patient sitting against the wall on the floor. He appears pale and his skin is dry. Pulse is 90; respirations are 18; blood pressure is 140/90.

26. You respond to a scene and find a young child who has just been pulled out of a cold stream. The child has no pulse and no respiration. You are told that the child had been in the stream for about 30 minutes.

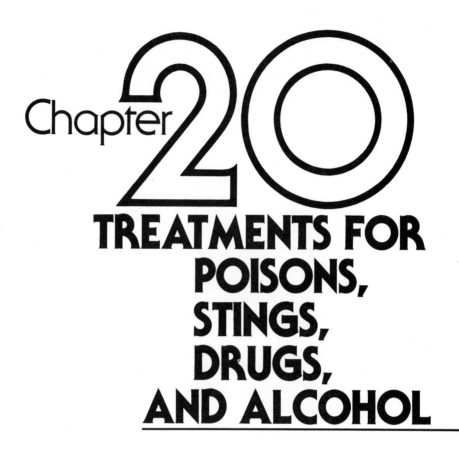

Chapter 20

TREATMENTS FOR POISONS, STINGS, DRUGS, AND ALCOHOL

Comprehensive Questions

1. What are the contraindications to inducing vomiting in a case of suspected or known poisoning? What are the reasons for these contraindications?

2. Why is dilution always a key step in the treatment of poisoning?

3. What is anaphylaxis? Describe the physiological changes which occur in a victim of anaphylactic shock and the clinical picture that is presented.

4. Why should a case of drug overdose be treated as a poisoning?

5. What is delirium tremens? Describe its clinical picture.

6. Describe the various ways that poisoning can occur.

7. Describe the procedure for treating a poisoning.

8. List the assumptions that the EMT must make when treating a poisoning.

Performance Skills

The proper treatment of poisoning, stings, and the abuse of drugs and alcohol requires the selection and application of many skills acquired at earlier stages of the course.

The primary new skill introduced here is the ability to recognize the various conditions that might present themselves and to select the proper treatment for them. These conditions include:

poisoning
snakebite
anaphylaxis
drug overdose
delirium tremens

Reference Data

1. **Signs and symptoms which may be present in a case of poisoning**
   a. nausea, vomiting
   b. abdominal pain
   c. diarrhea
   d. dilated or constricted pupils
   e. excess salivation
   f. diaphoresis
   g. abnormal respiration, cyanosis
   h. unconsciousness
   i. convulsions

2. To dilute poisons (using whole milk if possible)
   a. patients up to 100 pounds—one 8-ounce glass
   b. patients 101 to 150 pounds—one-and-a-half 8-ounce glasses
   c. patients over 150 pounds—two 8-ounce glasses

3. Never induce vomiting if the patient:
   a. is stuporous, semiconscious, or comatose
   b. has had convulsions

4. Never induce vomiting if the substance taken:
   a. is an acid or alkali
   b. has caused burns of the mouth, lips, or throat.

5. The EMT must always assume:
   a. that the substance taken is poisonous
   b. that the amount taken is toxic
   c. that the situation is life-threatening

6. **Clinical picture of anaphylaxis**
   a. severe itching with the presence of hives or inflamed skin
   b. swelling of the face with flushed, mottled, or ashen skin
   c. tightness of the chest with the feeling that the throat is closing up
   d. dyspnea, with sneezing, coughing, wheezing, or the coughing up of blood-tinged sputum
   e. rapid pulse with declining blood pressure
   f. abdominal cramps with nausea, vomiting, and diarrhea

Review Questions

Select the correct answer for each of the following questions. There is only *one* correct answer for each.

1. A patient has taken an overdose of a "downer." The EMT should:
    a. try to "talk him down."
    b. simply prevent the patient from injuring himself.
    c. maintain an airway and provide respiratory support.
    d. not be concerned since no life-threat exists.

2. The general treatment for poisoning when the patient is disoriented, stuporous, or unconscious is to:
    a. dilute, call poison control, and transport.
    b. treat for shock and call poison control.
    c. induce vomiting and call poison control.
    d. transport immediately to the nearest emergency room.

3. You are called for the third time to a house in which a teenager has twice before stated he swallowed a drug overdose. In both instances, he did not. The parents are certain no medication is missing. You should:
    a. call the police and request help in transporting "a patient."
    b. transport him immediately.
    c. begin treating for an ingested poison.

4. The constricting bands applied for a snakebite should:
    a. stop the flow of arterial blood, but not venous blood.
    b. stop the flow of venous blood, but not arterial blood.
    c. stop the flow of both arterial and venous blood.
    d. stop the capillary blood flow.

5. Anaphylactic shock is considered an emergency in:
    a. very few people.
    b. any patient.
    c. a sensitized person only.
    d. cases of bee sting only.

6. Which of the following groups of signs is indicative of shock?
    a. Slow, strong pulse; dizziness; cold perspiration; nausea.
    b. Rapid, weak pulse; cold, clammy skin; pallor; shallow breathing.
    c. Blank expression; cold extremities; regular breathing.
    d. Blank expression; chills; unconsciousness; dry skin.

7. Which of the following is *not* an indication of shock?
    a. Dull and lackluster eyes.
    b. Constricted pupils.
    c. Shallow respiration, possibly irregular or labored.
    d. Cold and clammy skin.

8. General treatment for poisoning when the patient is conscious and alert is to:
    a. dilute and call poison control.
    b. treat for shock and call poison control.
    c. induce vomiting and call poison control.
    d. transport immediately to the nearest emergency room.

9. Indicators of an anaphylactic reaction include:
    a. flushing, itching, or burning sensation to face and chest.
    b. pain, tightness, wheezing, and difficulty in breathing.
    c. falling BP, dizziness.
    d. all of the above.

10. Anaphylactic shock can be caused by:
    a. insect stings or bites.
    b. ingesting foods or drugs.
    c. injecting drugs.
    d. any of these.

11. You suspect that a conscious and alert patient has ingested an alkaline drain cleaner. Which would be most appropriate?
    a. Give vinegar to neutralize the alkali.
    b. Give ipecac and watch the airway.
    c. Give milk, then give ipecac, and call poison control.
    d. Dilute and call poison control.

12. A middle-aged woman with a known heart condition has taken an accidental overdose of a medication. She is alert and coherent. Of the following, your best course of action would be to:
    a. dilute and call poison control for instructions.
    b. dilute and induce vomiting.
    c. administer syrup of ipecac immediately.
    d. administer oxygen and transport.

13. A patient has been bitten by a snake and the extremity is swollen. You should:
    a. apply a venous constrictor above and below the site at the edge of the swelling.
    b. apply a venous constrictor above the site.
    c. apply a venous constrictor below the site.
    d. apply tourniquets above and below the site.

14. When giving emergency care to patients in shock, it is important to maintain adequate oxygen supply to the vital organs. To help in doing this, the EMT can:
    a. elevate the lower extremities, except in cases of head and chest injuries.
    b. slightly elevate the upper part of the body, except in cases of head and chest injuries.
    c. tilt the entire body down at the head.
    d. elevate the lower extremities and trunk of the body.

15. When treating patients in shock:
    a. oxygen should always be administered.
    b. oxygen is not an indicated treatment.
    c. oxygen is only an indicated treatment if respiratory difficulty or arrest occur.
    d. oxygen is only of peripheral benefit and should be administered after other treatment.

16. Carbon monoxide produces death by:
    a. over stimulating the central nervous system.
    b. destroying the alveoli of the lungs.
    c. combining with hemoglobin and reducing the amount of oxygen reaching body cells.
    d. combining with white blood cells and preventing oxygen from reaching body tissue.

17. You are called to a scene at which you find a sluggish and depressed patient who reportedly "took some drugs." His speech is slurred and he lacks physical coordination. You should suspect an overdose of:
    a. barbiturates.
    b. stimulants.
    c. hallucinogens.
    d. cocaine.

18. Plants can have a poisonous effect on the body because they may affect the:
    a. circulation.
    b. gastrointestinal tract.
    c. central nervous system.
    d. all of the above.

19. Syrup of ipecac should be used when treating a poison victim:
    a. regardless of circumstances.
    b. when no other means of treatment is available.
    c. when vomiting is required.
    d. when an acid has been ingested.

20. Unless contraindicated by other injuries, an unconscious patient of alcohol or drug abuse should be transported:
    a. on his back in the Trendelenberg position.
    b. on his back with both the head and foot portions of the cot elevated.
    c. on his back with his head elevated.
    d. on his side with his head lowered slightly.

21. When "talking down" an agitated patient, the EMT:
    a. attempts to instill confidence in the patient.
    b. is quiet, relaxed, and sympathetic.
    c. avoids physical restraints.
    d. all of the above.

22. Delirium tremens (DTs) may be indicated by:
    a. restlessness, fever, sweating.
    b. disorientation, confusion, delusions.
    c. hallucinations, agitation, wild behavior.
    d. any or all of these.

23. The course of treatment for the acutely intoxicated patient generally includes:
    a. treating for depression of the central nervous system.
    b. providing basic life support as required.
    c. survey carefully to locate all injuries.
    d. all of the above.

24. The EMT's attitude is important when treating an apparently drunken patient. Which of the following may be mistaken for intoxication?
    a. A diabetic emergency.
    b. A head injury.
    c. Epilepsy.
    d. All of these.

25. A patient suffering acute DTs can go into shock due to:
    a. a high percentage of alcohol in his blood.
    b. a loss of fluids caused by fever, sweating, and vomiting.
    c. convulsions.
    d. hallucinations.

26. When treating a patient for alcohol or drug abuse, the EMT should:
    a. maintain the patient's airway and prevent aspiration.
    b. prevent the patient from injuring himself.
    c. monitor the patient's level of consciousness.
    d. all of the above.

27. Alcohol, tranquilizers, barbiturates, and narcotics all:
    a. cause hallucinations.
    b. depress the central nervous system.
    c. present no life threat.
    d. are "uppers."

28. An EMT responds to a drug abuse call and finds the patient violent and incoherent. He says that he sees strange animals, and he tells the EMT that he can fly and wants to jump out the window. The EMT should suspect use of:
    a. barbiturates.
    b. stimulants.
    c. hallucinogens.
    d. heroin.

29. Delirium tremens (DTs) can be caused by:
    a. alcohol overdose.
    b. withdrawal from using alcohol.
    c. falling while intoxicated.
    d. all of the above.

30. A child has ingested an unknown number of leaves from a green houseplant. He is conscious and alert when you arrive. Of the following, your best course of action would be to:
    a. dilute, call poison control, request permission to induce vomiting.
    b. dilute, call poison control, request instructions.
    c. administer syrup of ipecac immediately.
    d. treat for shock and transport immediately.

Answers to Review Questions

1: c. "Downers" depress the central nervous system. The EMT should maintain an airway and provide respiratory support.

2: d. The EMT should treat this patient as a true emergency and transport immediately in the coma position.

3: c. The EMT must assume a toxic substance was taken and treat this patient for an ingested poison.

4: b. The constrictor should be tight enough to occlude venous return but not arterial flow.

5: b. Anaphylactic shock is a true emergency in any patient.

6: b. Rapid, weak pulse; cold, clammy skin; pallor; and shallow breathing are indicators of shock.

7: b. Constricted pupils are an indicator of the use of narcotics, not an indicator of shock.

8: a. With a conscious victim of poisoning, the EMT should dilute and call the poison control center.

9: d. All of these are indicators of an anaphylactic reaction.

10: d. Anaphylaxis can be caused by any of these.

11: d. Since this conscious patient ingested a substance not meant to be taken by mouth, the EMT should dilute with milk and call the poison control center for instructions.

12: a. The best course of action would be to dilute and call the poison control center for instructions.

13: b. The EMT should apply a venous constrictor above the site at the edge of the swelling.

14: a. The EMT should elevate the patient's lower extremities, except in cases of head and chest injuries.

15: a. Oxygen should be administered to all patients in shock.

16: c. Carbon monoxide combines with hemoglobin 200 times faster than does oxygen, so the amount of oxygen reaching body cells is reduced.

17: a. The symptoms indicate an overdose of barbiturates, or "downers."

18: d. All of these are effects that plants can have on the body.

19: c. Syrup of ipecac is used to induce vomiting.

20: d. An unconscious patient should be transported on his side with his head slightly lowered to aid in monitoring his airway.

21: d. The EMT should attempt to do all of these when trying to "talk down" a patient.

22: d. All of these are indicators of delirium tremens.

23: d. All of these should be included when treating an acutely intoxicated patient.

24: d. All of these conditions can be mistaken for intoxication.

25: b. The loss of fluids due to sweating, fever, and vomiting can cause the patient to go into shock.

26: d. All of these should be included in the treatment of a patient for alcohol or drug abuse.

27: b. All of these substances act to depress the central nervous system.

28: c. These symptoms indicate the use of a hallucinogen.

29: b. Delerium tremens may be caused by the sudden withdrawal from the use of alcohol.

30: a. The best course of action would be to dilute, call the poison control center, and request permission to induce vomiting.

Practical Applications

Consider how you would act, and why, in the following situations.

1. You respond to a motor vehicle accident. The only victim is a male of about 40 years who appears to be intoxicated. His only apparent injury is a minor scalp laceration. He is very abusive to you verbally and refuses treatment. The police officer in charge tells you to "get him out of here and take him to the hospital."

2. You are called to treat a 16-year-old female who appears to be covered with tiny, red, itchy welts. She recently has been under a doctor's care for a sore throat and has been taking penicillin. Her eyes appear swollen and she has difficulty breathing. Vitals are pulse 100; respiration 20; BP 110/70.

3. You respond to a house where a party is going on. A 16-year-old girl is found, unable to support herself and very groggy. According to friends she took some pills and had a little to drink. The type of pills and the quantity are not known.

4. You respond to a local park and find a derelict lying in the bushes. An empty wine bottle is next to him. He appears very groggy, is unable to support himself and seems to be uninjured. You detect a fruity smell on his breath.

5. A policeman reports that a car slowed down suddenly and came to a stop at the side of the road. The driver's window is open. The driver is unconscious and his face appears grotesquely swollen. He is barely breathing.

6. A young child at a family picnic was stung several times by a swarm of bees. The area where he was stung is red and swollen with several stingers imbedded in it. He complains of intense pain surrounding each sting. His parents tell you that he has no known allergic reaction to insect stings. His pulse is rapid.

7. You are called to a local high school where a teacher directs you to a youngster lying unconscious in a restroom. His left sleeve is rolled up and a rubber constricting band is secured just above the elbow. A syringe is found on the floor nearby. His blood pressure is 80/50; respirations are 6 and shallow; pulse is 20 and thready.

8. A 14-year-old boy who was playing on a hill behind his home has been bitten by an unidentified snake. He complains of severe burning pain and swelling around the fang marks on the back of his hand. As you treat him, he complains that the pain and swelling extend to his elbow. Vitals are: pulse, 110; respirations, 20; blood pressure, 100/70.

9. You are called to treat a 13-year-old boy who was camping out in the yard. When you arrive, the child is experiencing muscular cramps in his entire left arm with a burning pain. You notice 2 red dots just below the elbow, and there is discoloration and swelling. The child is sweating, complains of tightness across his chest, and seems to have trouble breathing. Vitals are: pulse, 100; respirations, 18 and labored; blood pressure, 100/70.

10. A small child has eaten tranquilizers and aspirin. You are unable to determine how many pills were taken or when.

11. While returning from a call, you notice a car pulled to the roadside with its parking lights on. The driver appears to be slumped over the steering wheel. He does not respond to direct questioning. A quick physical reveals slow respiration, slow pulse, and constricted pupils.

12. A toddler is found sitting on the kitchen floor crying and rubbing his stomach. Many leaves of a nearby houseplant are lying on the floor next to the child.

13. A child drank half a bottle of furniture polish and half a can of lighter fluid. The child is conscious.

14. You arrive to find that a woman, obviously pregnant, has taken a large number of capsules that were prescribed for her husband. She is conscious and calm.

15. A 4-year-old child has swallowed an unknown number of pills that were prescribed for the family's dog. When you arrive, he is conscious and coherent.

Chapter 21
PATIENT ASSESSMENT

Comprehensive Questions

1. Why must the primary survey be carried out first on all patients in all situations?

2. What are the things the EMT can learn almost immediately by simply looking at the patient? How does this help in the further assessment of the patient?

3. What injuries or conditions require you to discontinue your assessment and provide immediate treatment? Why?

4. Under what conditions would you package and transport a patient without conducting the full body pre-packaging survey?

5. Review in sequence and detail the steps involved in the thorough assessment of an emergency patient. At each step consider the possible signs and what each might indicate.

Performance Skills

The accurate assessment of a patient's condition requires many of the performance skills presented in earlier stages of the course. In particular, the skills listed in the chapter on diagnostic signs and patient examination must be carefully applied. It is the combination of these diagnostic skills with a thorough knowledge of medical concepts and conditions that allows for efficient, accurate patient assessment.

Reference Data

Sequence of Patient Assessment

1. Primary Assessment
   a. safety (yours and the patient's)
   b. observation
      1. mechanism; why called
      2. sex and approximate age of patient
      3. conscious or unconscious
      4. c-spine (Movement of the patient should be limited until it is determined that no spine injury is present.)
   c. breathing
      1. spontaneity of ventilation (presence, quality)
      2. patency of airway
      3. adequacy of air exchange (look, listen, feel)
   d. circulation
      1. pulse (presence, quality, regularity, estimation of blood pressure)
      2. skin color, temperature
      3. neck veins
   e. bleeding/deformity (Look for sites of major bleeding and marked deformity.)
   f. short CNS exam
      1. level of consciousness: *A*-alert; *V*-responds to verbal stimuli; *P*-responds to pain; *U*-unresponsive
      2. patient's ability to move
   g. major complaints
      1. history of this incident
      2. patient's name
   h. quality of ventilation and circulation—to include any or all, as needed:
      1. palpation of chest and trachea
      2. auscultation of chest
      3. percussion of chest
      4. blanching test
      5. inspection of mucosa of mouth
   i. support treatment or transport if necessary

Note: The primary assessment should take only 1-2 minutes.

2. Secondary Assessment
   a. Take respiratory and pulse rate, and blood pressure.
   b. Evaluate skin color and temperature.
   c. Record findings to this point.
   d. Evaluate any head, neck, or facial trauma.
   e. Examine abdomen and pelvis, if needed.
   f. Perform detailed CNS exam, if needed.
   g. Obtain history of this episode, past medical history, and the patient's personal data.

Note: Pertinent history will develop throughout the assessment as you talk to the patient or bystanders. With an unconscious patient be alert to look for Medi-Alert or wallet cards.

     h. Make other observations and perform diagnostic tests, as needed (based upon patient's condition, previous findings, or planned course of treatment).

     i. Review findings to be sure that the following have been eliminated:
   1. poisoning, drug overdose, anaphylaxis.
   2. hypoglycemia, diabetes, fasting, neglect.
   3. cardiac emergency.
   4. brain damage, CVA.
   5. contradictory findings.
   6. other possible patients.

     j. Treat all injuries and package for transport. Continue to monitor the patient and reassess as necessary.

Review Questions

Select the correct answer for each of the following questions. There is only *one* correct answer for each.

1. When examining an unconscious accident victim, check for injuries to an extremity by doing all of the following *except*:
    a. gently palpating the extremity.
    b. inspecting for deformity.
    c. manipulating the extremity for abnormal motion.
    d. checking pulse and sensation at the end of the extremity.

2. When surveying a scene involving one patient, the first thing the EMT should seek and react to is:
    a. possible bleeding.
    b. possible lack of breathing.
    c. possible danger of further accident or injury.
    d. possible neck or spine involvement.

3. The first priority of the primary survey is:
    a. identification of name and address of the patient.
    b. identification of life-threatening condition.
    c. identification of injuries that could cause permanent damage to the patient.
    d. all of the above.

4. If after the primary survey a bony protrusion in the patient's neck is discovered, the EMT should:
    a. stabilize the patient's head and neck before continuing the assessment.
    b. continue the assessment being careful not to move the patient's head.
    c. discontinue the assessment, place the patient on a stretcher, and transfer him immediately to a hospital.
    d. continue the assessment and then treat fractures before carrying out any other emergency care procedures.

5. An unconscious victim of an automobile accident is found slumped forward on the steering wheel. Your initial action, after making certain that you are not in any danger, should be to:
    a. establish and maintain axial traction.
    b. remove the victim from the automobile.
    c. establish an airway.
    d. establish the patient's vital signs.

6. In conducting the primary survey, use the following order:
    a. pulse, respiration, bleeding.
    b. respiration, bleeding, pulse.
    c. respiration, pulse, bleeding.
    d. pulse, bleeding, respiration.

7. EMTs should always check for bracelets or necklaces which:
   - a. give the patient's name and home address.
   - b. identify the patient's physician.
   - c. give the patient's social security number.
   - d. give information on medical problems.

8. While conducting his survey, the EMT notes the patient's skin condition. If a patient is in shock, the skin will appear:
   - a. cold, pale, moist.
   - b. cold, pale, dry.
   - c. hot, red, moist.
   - d. warm, pale, dry.

9. When presented with several patients, the EMT must determine an order of treatment based on the patients' conditions. This is known as:
   - a. survey.
   - b. triage.
   - c. placement.
   - d. analysis.

10. Arriving at a car wreck you find the driver impaled upon the steering column, one passenger with a fractured femur, and another passenger on the ground with dilated pupils. All 3 are hemorrhaging heavily from lacerations. You assign the driver:
    - a. first priority.
    - b. second priority.
    - c. third priority.

11. Upon arriving with the ambulance at a multi-patient accident, and determining that no additional danger to himself or others exists, the EMT should then:
    - a. treat the patient who is the most seriously injured.
    - b. survey all patients to ascertain the extent of injury to each.
    - c. treat whoever is bleeding.
    - d. treat women and children first.

12. Which would you suspect if you saw a broken steering wheel?
    - a. Whiplash.
    - b. Fractured femur.
    - c. Fractured tibia.
    - d. Flail chest.

13. To survey for paralysis in a conscious patient, you should first:
    - a. touch the wrists and ankles and ask for a response.
    - b. have the patient lift his arms.
    - c. have the patient move his fingers.
    - d. have the patient grasp your hand.

14. The abdomen is divided into how many sections for the purpose of communication, organ location, and diagnosis?
    a. 2.
    b. 4.
    c. 6.
    d. 8.

15. Pain and tenderness in the upper right quadrant of the abdomen, without trauma, often indicates:
    a. ruptured spleen.
    b. appendicitis.
    c. gallbladder disease.
    d. disease of the kidney.

16. Pain and tenderness in the lower right quadrant of the abdomen often indicates:
    a. ruptured spleen.
    b. appendicitis.
    c. gallbladder disease.
    d. disease of the kidney.

17. Pain and tenderness in the upper left quadrant of the abdomen often indicates:
    a. ruptured spleen.
    b. appendicitis.
    c. gallbladder disease.
    d. injury to the ureter.

18. Which one of the following measures is *not* part of the *primary* survey of an accident victim?
    a. Checking for a pulse.
    b. Checking for a ruptured spleen.
    c. Checking for severe bleeding.
    d. Checking for signs of breathing.

19. An unconscious patient is making a snoring noise when he breathes. The EMT should suspect that the patient:
    a. is suffering from an MI.
    b. has a partially obstructed airway.
    c. is intoxicated.
    d. has a sucking chest wound.

20. You are called to a bar where a person is found on the floor. He is semi-conscious and appears to be intoxicated. You should:
    a. tell the patient to go home and sleep it off.
    b. get bystanders to take the patient home.
    c. call the police, and return to your station.
    d. make a thorough assessment of the patient and transport to the emergency department.

21. A palpable carotid pulse on one side but *not* on the other is an indicator of:
    a. cardiac arrest.
    b. cerebrovascular accident.
    c. myocardial infarction.
    d. occlusion of that carotid artery.

22. An EMT finds an unconscious woman. After making certain that neither he nor the patient is in danger, his first step in caring for this patient is to:
    a. force air into her lungs.
    b. determine her responsiveness.
    c. tilt her head back.
    d. check for a pulse.

23. In order to determine the extent of injury of an unconscious patient, the EMT should:
    a. listen to statements of bystanders.
    b. observe the patient's obvious injuries.
    c. observe injury-producing mechanisms.
    d. all of the above.

24. Which of the following is a life-threatening condition that requires the immediate attention of the EMT?
    a. Neck fractures.
    b. Fluid from the ears.
    c. Severe bleeding.
    d. All of the above.

25. A patient cannot respond to your touching his arms or legs; cannot wiggle his toes or fingers; cannot raise his legs or arms. What conclusions should you reach?
    a. Patient probably has a spinal cord injury below the neck.
    b. Patient probably has an injury in the cervical area.
    c. Patient probably does not have a spinal cord injury.
    d. Patient probably has a brain tumor.

26. A patient in an automobile wreck has no feeling below the level of the clavicle. You should suspect injury to the:
    a. cervical spine.
    b. thoracic spine.
    c. lumbar spine.
    d. sacral spine.

27. Which one of the following is *not* part of the primary survey?
    a. Checking for a CVA.
    b. Checking for a severe hemorrhage.
    c. Checking for an airway.
    d. Checking for a pulse.

28. Skin color is a diagnostic sign. A pale, white, ashen color may be indicative of:
    a. carbon monoxide poisoning.
    b. insufficient circulation or shock.
    c. lack of oxygen.
    d. jaundice.

29. The respiratory quality and rate of a patient in shock is likely to be:
    a. shallow and rapid.
    b. barely perceptible.
    c. shallow and slow.
    d. deep and rapid.

30. The quality and rate of the pulse of a patient in shock is likely to be:
    a. weak and slow.
    b. bounding and slow.
    c. weak and rapid.
    d. bounding and rapid.

31. Pupils of unequal size may indicate:
    a. cardiac or respiratory arrest.
    b. drug addiction or central nervous disease.
    c. myopia.
    d. Increased intracranial pressure.

32. A bluish-gray tint to the skin is an indication of:
    a. high blood pressure.
    b. diabetic coma.
    c. carbon monoxide poisoning.
    d. asphyxia.

33. A patient complains of numbness or tingling in both his legs. You should suspect an injury to:
    a. those limbs.
    b. the head.
    c. the spinal cord.
    d. the pelvis.

34. Absence of respiration and both carotid pulses usually indicates:
    a. shock.
    b. brain injury.
    c. cardiac arrest.
    d. stroke.

35. Red skin is an indication of:
    a. shock.
    b. carbon monoxide poisoning.
    c. cyanosis.
    d. frostbite.

36. Markedly constricted pupils tend to indicate:
    a. a cerebrovascular accident.
    b. cardiac arrest or respiratory arrest.
    c. a head injury.
    d. narcotic abuse.

37. Pupils that are equal but widely dilated tend to indicate:
    a. an anxious or unconscious state, cardiac arrest, or death.
    b. a neck injury.
    c. the use of narcotics.
    d. a cerebrovascular accident.

Answers to Review Questions

1: c. A limb or extremity should not be manipulated by the EMT.

2: c. The potential for further accident or injury must always be eliminated as soon as possible.

3: b. The purpose of the primary survey is to identify life-threatening conditions.

4: a. The secondary survey should be interrupted until the patient's neck and head have been stabilized.

5: c. You should always establish and maintain an airway first.

6: c. The sequence of the primary survey is airway (spontaneous ventilation), circulation, bleeding.

7: d. Many people with special problems wear bracelets or necklaces naming a medical condition, *e.g.*, "diabetic," "allergic to penicillin."

8: a. A patient in shock usually appears cold, pale, and moist.

9: b. Triage refers to the screening and classification of the sick or injured to determine priorities of treatment.

10: c. The salvage potential of the driver is very low due to the apparent severity of his injuries. Treating him first may cause the unnecessary death of one of the others.

11: b. You should quickly survey *all* victims to establish priority of treatment.

12: d. A flail chest or other thoracic injury should be suspected if impact was great enough to cause the steering wheel to break.

13: a. First touch the patient's extremities and ask if he feels your hands.

14: b. The abdomen is divided into 4 quadrants. The right and left upper quadrants, and the right and left lower quadrants.

15: c. Pain in the upper right quadrant may indicate gallbladder disease.

16: b. Tenderness and pain in the lower right quadrant may indicate appendicitis.

17: a. A ruptured spleen is often indicated by pain in the upper left quadrant.

18: b. The primary survey determines if there is spontaneous respiration, spontaneous circulation, and severe hemorrhage.

19: b. A snoring sound is indicative of an obstructed airway.

20: d. An intoxicated patient should be treated the same as any other patient.

21: d. The absence of one carotid pulse indicates occlusion of that artery.

22: b. Determining the responsiveness of the patient is always the first step in the primary survey of an apparently unconscious patient.

23: d. All of these items contribute to the EMT's complete assessment of the patient.

24: c. The control of severe bleeding requires immediate action.

25: b. The EMT should suspect and treat for a cord injury of the cervical spine.

26: b. The nerves of the cervical spine end at the clavicle; therefore the loss of sensation below the clavicle indicates thoracic injury.

27: a. The goal of the primary survey is to find out if the patient is breathing, hemorrhaging, and has adequate circulation.

28: b. A pale or ashen skin color indicates poor circulation, or shock.

29: a. Shallow and rapid respirations are indicators of shock.

30: c. The pulse of a patient in shock is usually weak and rapid.

31: d. Increased intracranial pressure.

32: d. Cyanosis is caused by low oxygen saturation of hemoglobin.

33: c. Numbness or tingling in the legs is an indicator of injury to the spinal cord.

34: c. These symptoms occurring together are indicators of cardiac arrest.

35: b. Red skin is an indicator of carbon monoxide poisoning.

36: d. Constricted pupils ("pinpoint") indicate the use of narcotics.

37: a. Equal but widely dilated pupils indicate the conditions described.

Practical Applications

Consider how you would conduct your assessment in each of the following situations.

1. You are called to assist a middle-aged man complaining of severe chest pains. You find him sitting in a living room chair.

2. You are called to a local bar where there has been a fight. A man about 30 years old is found unconscious on the floor, bleeding severely from a knife wound in his chest.

3. You are called to assist an elderly man with "difficulty in breathing." The patient is found in his bed, conscious but unwilling to communicate because of his breathing difficulty.

4. A woman in her 30s collapses in a shopping mall. When you arrive she is on the floor, unconscious, with her head in a friend's lap.

5. You are called to assist a man that was "hurt while cutting wood." When you arrive, you find a man in his 40s, sitting against a tree stump, holding his blood-soaked thigh. There is a chain saw at his feet. He is conscious and apparently in pain.

6. A young man's right leg is pinned under his motorcycle. It is severely angulated. He is conscious and communicative.

7. A woman has taken an *apparent* overdose of a prescribed medication. She is unconscious on the bathroom floor. Upon checking, you find there are no respirations.

8. A man's hand has been amputated at the wrist in an industrial accident. There is severe bleeding from the stump.

9. A high school student has been injured in a football game. He is wearing full equipment and complaining that it hurts when he breathes.

10. The driver of a car that was involved in an accident with another car appears to be unconscious, and his head is resting on his right shoulder.

For each of the following situations, assess the patients and categorize them in order of their priority of treatment.

11. You respond to a 2-car accident. Both cars are upright. The driver of car #1 is unconscious and secured to the seat with a seat belt. The head of the passenger in the front seat has smashed through the windshield. He is bleeding profusely about the face and neck and is unconscious. The driver of car #2 is wandering around

moaning "Oh, no." The passenger of car #2 is seated in the front seat, is sweating, and appears to be short of breath. He complains of severe chest pain and pain in his left arm. Another passenger is found lying in the road moaning that she cannot move her legs.

12. You arrive at the scene of an accident and find a driver and one passenger in the vehicle. Both are fastened in their seat belts. The driver is coughing up bright, frothy blood and is barely conscious. The passenger is unconscious and has lacerations of the scalp. His respirations are 12 and shallow; pulse is 120 and weak; bloody fluid is dripping from his nose and ears.

13. You are called to a one-car accident. You find the driver unconscious. He is fastened in his seat belt and there is dark red blood oozing from his mouth. The passenger in the back seat has an open fracture of the left tibia and is bleeding profusely at the fracture site.

14. You are first on the scene of a school bus-car accident. The bus has 12 elementary school students; the car has 2 adults.

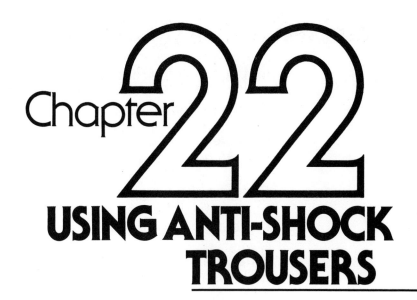

Chapter 22
USING ANTI-SHOCK TROUSERS

Comprehensive Questions

1. List and describe the three basic physiological conditions which cause hypotension (regardless of what illness or injury initiates the condition).

2. Why are a clinical picture of shock *and* a blood pressure below 90 mm Hg *both* required for anti-shock trousers to be indicated?

3. Describe the way in which the circumferential counterpressure applied by inflated anti-shock trousers affects the circulatory system.

4. What are the relative contraindications (conditions which *may* make use inappropriate) for anti-shock trousers? What should you do if one of these conditions is present?

5. What are the relative contraindications for the use of the abdominal section of anti-shock trousers?

6. Describe how you would examine a patient for the existence of pulmonary edema. What are the signs of this condition?

7. Besides combatting shock, what other beneficial effects can anti-shock trousers provide?

8. Why should anti-shock trousers never be deflated in the field?

Performance Skills

1. Assess a patient to determine if anti-shock trousers are indicated, and if any relative contraindications are present.

2. Prepare anti-shock trousers so they are protected from punctures or tears.

3. Apply anti-shock trousers to a patient and inflate them to the proper level.

4. Properly move a patient with anti-shock trousers onto the ambulance cot.

5. Maintain the inflation of a section of the anti-shock trousers should a leak occur.

Reference Data

1. Anti-shock trousers should only be used under medical direction.

2. **Indications:**
   The use of anti-shock trousers is indicated for any patient in shock when:
   a. a clinical picture of shock is present, and
   b. systolic blood pressure is below 90 mm Hg.
   Both *a* and *b* must be present for anti-shock trousers to be indicated.

3. **Contraindications:** There are no *absolute* contraindications to the use of anti-shock trousers.

4. **Relative contraindications:** The use of anti-shock trousers *may* be inappropriate if any of the following conditions are present:
   a. pulmonary edema
   b. cardiogenic shock; cardiac arrest from any cause other than hypovolemia

5.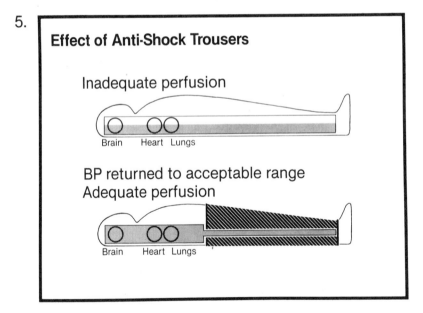

6. **Relative contraindications for abdominal section:** The following conditions may cause use of the abdominal section to be inappropriate treatment:
   a. pregnancy beyond the first trimester
   b. abdominal evisceration
   c. barbed or markedly irregular object impaled in abdomen (physician may order the removal of an impaled object with a smooth surface and the application of the garment)

7. The directing physician must be specifically told of any sign that might indicate a relative contraindication. It will be his decision to either withhold the garment or override the contraindication.

8. Anti-shock trousers should be inflated only until the patient's blood pressure has returned to 100 to 110 mm Hg, or the suit is at maximum pressure.

9. Anti-shock trousers should never be deflated in the field.

10. Anti-shock trousers should never be rapidly deflated under any circumstances.

Review Questions

Select the correct answer for each of the following questions. There is only *one* correct answer for each.

1. Anti-shock trousers can stabilize BP within a range of:
   a. 30 to 50 mm Hg systolic.
   b. 50 to 70 mm Hg systolic.
   c. 70 to 90 mm Hg systolic.
   d. 90 to 110 mm Hg systolic.

2. Anti-shock trousers should be applied so that the upper margin:
   a. lies across the pelvic girdle.
   b. is about 1 inch below the 12th rib.
   c. is at the level of the patient's nipples.
   d. is just below the xiphoid process.

3. A change in environmental temperature after anti-shock trousers have been inflated:
   a. will have no effect on the pressure within the suit.
   b. may cause the pressure within the suit to change.
   c. will cause the patient's condition to deteriorate.
   d. should be reported to the emergency department.

4. Once inflated, anti-shock trousers should be deflated:
   a. at the emergency department after definitive treatment has been initiated.
   b. after 30 minutes, then reinflated.
   c. by the emergency department triage nurse.
   d. at the emergency department by the ambulance crew so they will be prepared for the next call.

5. A disadvantage of anti-shock trousers is that once applied:
   a. the patient cannot move.
   b. the patient cannot receive IV fluids.
   c. a blood pressure cannot be taken.
   d. examination of the abdomen is limited.

6. Anti-shock trousers can autotransfuse:
   a. 2 units (1000 ml).
   b. 1 unit (500 ml).
   c. ½ unit (250 ml).
   d. between ¼ and ⅓ units (125 to 335 ml).

7. The EMT should take the patient's blood pressure before requesting permission to inflate anti-shock trousers, and again:
   a. between each step of inflation.
   b. before transporting the patient.
   c. while enroute to the emergency department.
   d. all of the above.

8. An adult male patient is said to be hypotensive when the clinical picture of shock is present *and* his systolic blood pressure is at or below:
   a. 90.
   b. 110.
   c. 130.
   d. 150.

9. The use of anti-shock trousers may be inappropriate with a patient who has:
   a. intracranial bleeding.
   b. intrathoracic bleeding.
   c. pulmonary edema.
   d. all of the above.

10. The EMT must contact the emergency department and advise the physician that a shock patient has a condition where the use of anti-shock trousers may be inappropriate because:
    a. the physician may wish to order the inflation of the suit in spite of this condition.
    b. he will need it for his report.
    c. additional manpower will be required in the field.
    d. higher pressure in the suit may be required under these conditions.

11. The EMT should begin basic treatment for shock on a patient who may be a candidate for anti-shock trousers:
    a. as soon as this condition is suspected.
    b. after receiving permission from the emergency room.
    c. after the patient has been placed in the suit.
    d. after the suit has been inflated.

12. The leg sections of anti-shock trousers should be inflated before the other sections:
    a. because most candidates for the trousers have severe leg injuries.
    b. so that blood is pushed toward the vital organs.
    c. because they are connected directly to the foot pump.
    d. because the suit is designed for use this way.

13. Once the blood pressure of a patient in anti-shock trousers has reached an acceptable level, the pressure within the suit:
    a. should be increased by 20 mm Hg as a safety margin.
    b. should be maintained at whatever pressure resulted in the acceptable systolic pressure.
    c. should be decreased by 20 mm Hg.
    d. should be adjusted so that the abdomen is 20 mm Hg lower than the legs.

14. What is the relationship between the readings of the suit gauge (or gauges) and the patient's blood pressure?
    a. The suit gauges measure the patient's systolic blood pressure in each leg and the abdomen.
    b. The suit gauges measure diastolic pressure only.
    c. The suit gauges will tell the EMT when the patient's blood pressure has reached an acceptable level.
    d. There is no relationship between the suit gauge readings and the patient's blood pressure.

15. The amount of pressure within anti-shock trousers required to cause a patient's blood pressure to reach an acceptable range:
    a. will rarely be more than 30 mm Hg.
    b. will rarely be more than 50 mm Hg.
    c. will usually be the maximum of that particular suit.
    d. cannot be predicted in advance.

16. Anti-shock trousers are of value in treating a patient with:
    a. a traumatic amputation of a lower limb.
    b. an abdominal aneurysm.
    c. a fractured pelvis.
    d. all of the above.

17. As part of the assessment for determining a patient's candidacy for anti-shock trousers, the EMT should:
    a. assess lung sounds.
    b. determine body weight.
    c. suction the oropharynx thoroughly.
    d. insert an oropharyngeal airway.

18. Anti-shock trousers:
    a. can serve as inflatable splints for lower extremities.
    b. will control internal bleeding in the abdomen and leg.
    c. force available blood from the portions of the body enclosed by the inflated segments to the heart and other vital organs.
    d. all of the above.

19. The measure of the successful use of MAST is:
    a. whether the patient survives.
    b. when the patient's systolic pressure increases.
    c. when the suit is fully inflated.
    d. when cyanosis disappears.

20. Anti-shock trousers may be of value in treating a patient:
    a. with a fractured femur.
    b. with a suspected ruptured spleen.
    c. with a gunshot wound to the abdomen.
    d. all of the above.

Answers to Review Questions

1: d. A patient's systolic blood pressure will usually stabilize within the range of 90 to 110 mm Hg.

2: b. The upper margin of the garment should be approximately 1 inch below the rib cage so as not to restrict respiration.

3: b. A change in temperature may cause the pressure within the suit to change.

4: a. Anti-shock trousers should only be deflated after definitive medical treatment has been started.

5: d. Once anti-shock trousers have been inflated, the portion of the body enclosed within them cannot be seen or palpated.

6: a. Anti-shock trousers can autotransfuse at least 2 units of the patient's own blood.

7: d. The patient's blood pressure should be taken at all of these stages of pre-hospital care.

8: a. A systolic blood pressure of 90 mm Hg is considered to be the threshold of shock according to many protocols, as long as the other indicators of shock are present.

9: c. The use of anti-shock trousers may be inappropriate with pulmonary edema.

10: a. The physician can override any contraindication and order the garment to be inflated.

11: a. The EMT should begin to treat a patient for shock as soon as that condition is suspected.

12: b. The leg sections are inflated first so that blood is "milked" from the legs and pushed toward the viscera.

13: b. Once a patient's blood pressure has reached an acceptable level, the pressure in the suit must be maintained at the pressure that caused the blood pressure to become stabilized.

14: d. There is no relationship between the readings of the suit gauges and the patient's blood pressure.

15: d. The amount of pressure within the suit that will be required to stabilize a patient's blood pressure within an acceptable range cannot be predicted in advance.

16: d. Anti-shock trousers are of value in all of these conditions.

17: a. The EMT should listen to the patient's lungs for the presence of moist rales indicating pulmonary edema.

18: d. All of these are functions of anti-shock trousers.

19: b. The successful use of MAST can be determined if the patient's systolic blood pressure returns to 100 to 110 mm Hg.

20: d. Anti-shock trousers are of value in all of these conditions.

Practical Applications

Consider how you would act, and why, in the following situations.

1. An adult male has been hit by a car while jogging. He is unconscious, has minor facial lacerations, and a possible fractured femur. Vital signs are: pulse, 140 and weak; blood pressure, 84/50; pupils, equal but slow to react; skin color, ashen; skin temperature, cool; respirations, 32 and rapid.

2. A middle-aged female is found unconscious at her home. There is a history of diabetes. Vital signs are: pulse, 130 and thready; blood pressure, 74 by palpation; respirations, 40 and deep; skin, dry and flushed; pupils, equal and sluggish.

3. A teenage female is unconscious in a chair. You are told she took some pills and drank an undetermined amount of whiskey. Vital signs are: pulse, 166 and weak; blood pressure, 58 by palpation; respirations, 10 and shallow.

4. An adult male was involved in a collision with a car while riding his motorcycle, and was thrown 50 feet from the point of impact. You find the patient conscious, on his back. Open fractures of the left femur and right tibia-fibula are evident as well as superficial lacerations to the arms and legs. He does not complain of back pain, but there is significant pain in the right and left upper quadrants. Palpation of the abdomen reveals guarding and tenderness. Visual examination shows abrasions and contusions of the lower chest and upper abdomen. Vital signs are: pulse, 150; blood pressure, 86/44; respirations, rapid.

5. A man has been shot in the chest after an argument in a bar. You find him unconscious on his back. Hemorrhage is severe. There is no exit wound. Carotid pulses are barely palpable, and respirations are 28. Blood pressure is 60 by palpation.

6. A man has suffered third-degree burns to both legs, abdomen, and chest in an industrial accident. Your assessment indicates a systolic blood pressure of 82; pulse of 120; respirations of 32; pupils equal.

7. You respond to an industrial accident to find a man with his hand caught in a machine. He is unconscious and is being supported in a standing position by 2 co-workers. They tell you it will take almost 5 minutes to free their friend's hand. Vitals are: pulse, 120; blood pressure, 78/42; respirations, 42.

8. A man has been shot in the thigh with an arrow in a hunting accident. It occurred 20 minutes ago and the arrow is still impaled in his thigh. Vitals are: systolic pressure, 140/90; pulse, 120.

9. You are called to assist a middle-aged man with severe dyspnea. When you arrive he is sitting upright in a chair. He reports that he suffered a heart attack 8 months ago. He denies pain. Vitals are: pulse, 130; blood pressure, 100/60; he is diaphoretic.

10. The driver of a car involved in a motor vehicle accident is conscious when you arrive. Your assessment indicates no apparent lacerations, full reaction to painful stimuli, no suspicion of fractures. He tells you that he did not hit his head, did not lose consciousness, but has pain in his abdomen where he hit the steering wheel, and that he suffered "whiplash." Initial vital signs are: pulse, 94; blood pressure, 110/70; respirations, 40.

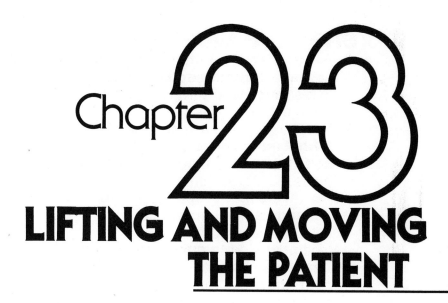

Chapter 23

LIFTING AND MOVING THE PATIENT

Comprehensive Questions

1. What are the acceptable methods for lifting a patient from the floor or ground to an ambulance cot? What are the advantages and disadvantages of each?

2. What are the acceptable methods for transferring a patient from a bed to an ambulance cot?

3. What are the acceptable methods for transferring a patient from a chair to an ambulance cot?

4. What are the common devices available to the EMT for carrying a patient? What are the advantages, disadvantages, and contraindications of each?

5. What are the factors the EMT must consider before choosing a method of lifting and moving the patient?

6. Why should the stair chair not usually be used to carry an unconscious patient down stairs?

Performance Skills

1. Transfer a patient directly from a bed to an ambulance cot.

2. Transfer a patient directly from a chair to an ambulance cot.

3. Lift a patient from the floor or ground to an ambulance cot:
   a. using a blanket lift.
   b. using a split litter.
   c. using a long backboard.

4. Lift and carry a patient down a flight of stairs:
   a. using a stair chair.
   b. using a long backboard.
   c. using a split litter.

5. Safely raise, lower, roll, load, and unload an ambulance cot.

6. Transfer a patient from an ambulance cot to an emergency room table.

7. Safely pass a split litter, backboard, or Stokes litter over a wall or fence.

8. Safely pass a Stokes litter up a steep incline.

9. Quickly remove a patient from a hostile environment using a body drag.

Reference Data

1. Factors in choosing method of lifting and moving
   a. patient's medical condition
   b. treatment being given
   c. need for rapid transportation
   d. environmental situation
   e. number of responders available

2. Devices available for lifting and moving
   a. split litter
   b. long backboard
   c. stair chair
   d. Stokes basket litter
   e. ambulance cot

3. Contraindications for stair chair
   a. spine injury
   b. fracture of lower extremity
   c. most unconscious patients

4. Contraindications for split litter
   a. spine injury
   b. patient with anti-shock trousers (MAST)

5. Basic principles of lifting
   a. keep the device close to your body
   b. avoid leaning or stretching
   c. lift with your legs, not your back
   d. place hands under device, palms up
   e. avoid twisting your trunk
   f. keep feet placed one in front of the other for support

Review Questions

Select the correct answer for each of the following questions. There is only *one* correct answer for each.

1. Which of the following methods would you use to move a patient from the vicinity of a possible explosion?
    a. Place him on a split litter.
    b. Place him in a stair chair.
    c. Drag him along the long axis of his body.
    d. Secure him to a backboard with cravats.

2. When lifting a litter, you should avoid:
    a. lifting with your legs, not your back.
    b. twisting the trunk of your body.
    c. keeping one foot in front of the other.
    d. placing hands palms up under the litter.

3. Which of the following should the EMT do first if he plans to use a chair to carry a patient down a flight of stairs?
    a. Test the chair for sturdiness.
    b. Tilt the chair backwards.
    c. Restrain the patient's arms and legs.
    d. Place the patient's hands in his lap.

4. Before moving a patient, the EMT should consider:
    a. if the patient is in immediate danger.
    b. if there is a suspected spinal injury.
    c. what help is available.
    d. all of the above.

5. An efficient method of moving a patient from a bed to the ambulance cot is the:
    a. blanket slide.
    b. 2-man seat carry.
    c. 2-man pickup.
    d. pack-strap carry.

6. Which of the following devices should be used to move a patient over rough terrain or from heights?
    a. Stokes basket.
    b. Split-frame stretcher.
    c. Ambulance cot.
    d. Split litter.

7. A disadvantage of the split litter is that:
    a. it must be separated before using.
    b. both sides of the patient must be accessible.
    c. it comes in only one length.
    d. 2 EMTs are required to use it.

8. An unconscious patient should generally be positioned on the ambulance cot:
    a. in a prone position.
    b. in a supine position.
    c. on his side.
    d. in a semi-sitting position.

9. Which of the following devices should be used to transport an unconscious patient down stairs?
    a. Split litter or full backboard.
    b. Split litter or stair chair.
    c. Stair chair or backboard.
    d. Stair chair or ambulance cot.

10. Which of the following is the least effective device to transport a patient down a flight of stairs from an upper floor?
    a. Split litter.
    b. Backboard.
    c. Stair chair.
    d. Ambulance cot.

11. A conscious patient suspected of having a cardiac episode in an upper floor bedroom should be:
    a. asked to walk slowly down the stairs to the ambulance cot.
    b. placed in a stair chair and carried down.
    c. placed in a Stokes basket and lowered out the window.
    d. carried down the stairs by two EMTs using the extremity carry.

12. Both the straddle slide and log-roll are techniques used to:
    a. place a patient onto a backboard.
    b. transport a patient safely.
    c. splint a patient effectively.
    d. place a patient on the ambulance cot.

13. To protect the integrity of the patient's spinal cord, the log-roll technique should *not* be attempted unless how many EMTs are available?
    a. 2.
    b. 3.
    c. 4.
    d. 5.

14. How many EMTs are required to straddle slide a patient onto a backboard?
    a. 2.
    b. 3.
    c. 4.
    d. 5.

15. A patient in a Stokes basket must be moved up a steep hill. The EMTs should:
    a. pass the patient along.
    b. walk up the hill supporting the basket with one hand.
    c. walk up the hill sideways with both hands on the basket.
    d. all of the above are acceptable.

16. If an accident victim must be moved to safety, he should be:
    a. moved using the fireman's carry.
    b. pulled along the long axis of the body.
    c. secured to a backboard.
    d. carried in the EMT's arms.

17. A patient can be placed in the shock position on the ambulance cot by raising the Trendelenberg lift and:
    a. elevating the head portion until his head is higher than his heart.
    b. placing a pillow under his feet.
    c. elevating the head portion until his head and trunk are parallel to the frame of the cot.
    d. placing a pillow under his head.

18. When using a split litter:
    a. both halves should be separated to place it under the patient.
    b. only the foot end need be separated.
    c. only the head end need be separated.
    d. all of the above are acceptable.

19. An ambulance crew has brought the cot up 5 or 6 stairs into a patient's home. The patient is receiving oxygen and is sitting upright on the cot. The cot should be carried down the stairs:
    a. head first.
    b. feet first.
    c. by no less than 3 EMTs.
    d. by no less than 4 EMTs.

20. A patient that is secured to a split litter should be carried down a flight of stairs:
    a. head first.
    b. feet first.
    c. tilted to one side.
    d. by no less than 4 EMTs.

21. To avoid injuring himself while lifting a patient, the EMT should:
    a. use one hand.
    b. always use both hands.
    c. lift from his legs, not with his back.
    d. bend over so he lifts with his back.

22. A patient that has been immobilized onto a backboard can be placed in the shock position by:
    a. the Trendelenberg lift.
    b. elevating the head portion.
    c. positioning him on his side.
    d. using the "contour" crank.

23. A patient's respirations can be affected when he is placed in the Trendelenberg position because:
    a. his head is higher than his heart.
    b. he is on his side.
    c. the abdominal organs may press against his diaphragm.
    d. his knees are flexed.

Answers to Review Questions

1: c. A patient should be moved from a hostile environment as quickly as possible using a body drag.

2: b. You should avoid twisting the trunk of your body when lifting any device.

3: a. The chair should be tested for sturdiness before the patient is placed on it.

4: d. The EMT should take all of these factors into consideration before moving a patient.

5: a. The blanket slide is an easy method of moving a patient from a bed to an ambulance cot.

6: a. The Stokes basket should be used in these situations.

7: b. A disadvantage of the split litter is that there must be room on both sides of the patient so the litter halves can be placed under him.

8: c. An unconscious patient should be placed on his side so that his airway can be properly maintained.

9: a. An unconscious patient should be properly secured to a split litter or a backboard to be safely transported down a flight of stairs.

10: d. Due to its weight and bulk, the ambulance cot is the least effective device.

11: b. A conscious patient should be placed in a stair chair and carried down the stairs.

12: a. Both these techniques are used to place a patient onto a long board.

13: c. Four EMTs are required to perform the log roll.

14: c. Four EMT's are required to perform the straddle slide.

15: a. The Stokes basket should be passed along. As each EMT passes the basket, he moves to the front to receive it again.

16: b. An accident victim should be pulled along the long axis of his body.

17: c. The head portion should be raised until the patient's head and trunk are parallel to the frame of the cot.

18: a. The halves of the litter must be separated before a patient can be placed on it.

19: a. The patient should be carried head first in this situation to maintain both his position and stability on the ambulance cot.

20: b. The patient secured to a split litter or backboard should be carried feet first down the stairs.

21: c. The EMT should always lift from his legs, never from his back.

22: a. A patient on a backboard can be placed in the shock position by elevating the Trendelenberg lift.

23: c. The Trendelenberg position can impair a patient's respirations by causing the abdominal organs to press against the diaphragm.

Practical Applications

Describe how you would transfer the patient to the ambulance cot in each of the following situations.

1. You respond with another EMT to find an unconscious adult male in a bed on the second floor of a 2-level home. There is no indication of either spinal injury or fractures.

2. A child riding his bicycle has been hit by a car. He is unconscious. Your assessment indicates suspected fractures of the right radius and ulna, and left tibia and fibula. You apply splints to both affected extremities.

3. You respond to a private home to find an elderly female in respiratory distress. Your assessment includes swelling of the ankles and a history of a previous cardiac emergency. She is sitting upright in a living room chair. You decide to bring the ambulance cot into the room.

4. A child has fallen from a skateboard. She is conscious, in pain, and very frightened. Your assessment notes pain in the right leg, a yellowish fluid collecting in her right ear, and black and blue marks and swelling under her eyes.

5. A young man has been lost in the woods and has been the subject of an extensive search operation. He is found unconscious, about 2 miles from the nearest road.

6. You suspect that a patient found conscious and sitting up in a bed on the second floor of his home is having a cardiac episode. You begin to administer oxygen by mask.

7. A very tall and obese male has collapsed in his backyard. He is found unconscious and on his side. A police officer is on the scene when you arrive with another EMT. You decide to bring the ambulance cot next to the patient.

8. A female patient is found in a semi-conscious state in her bed on the first floor of a private home. You bring the cot up the outside steps, into the bedroom, and alongside the bed.

9. An elderly man is found unconscious on the floor of a small bathroom on the second floor of his home. He is on his side, wedged between the bowl and bathtub. You suspect he is suffering a diabetic emergency. There is no indication of any fracture.

10. A woman has fallen down a flight of stairs. When you arrive she is sitting on the floor with her back against the wall. She tells you that both her right ankle and knee are very painful and that she cannot stand up. There is enough room to bring the ambulance cot near her.

11. You arrive at an auto accident to find a patient lying on the road near the rear of the car. He is unconscious and lying on his side. Gasoline is leaking from the car and pooling under his left leg.

12. You arrive at an office building and find a patient in an office at the end of a long corridor on the twenty-second floor. The patient is complaining of severe chest pains. He's diaphoretic and anxious.

13. You respond to a home. The patient is in the basement. You determine that he has fallen and has a fractured femur. The only exit from the basement is up a narrow stairway.

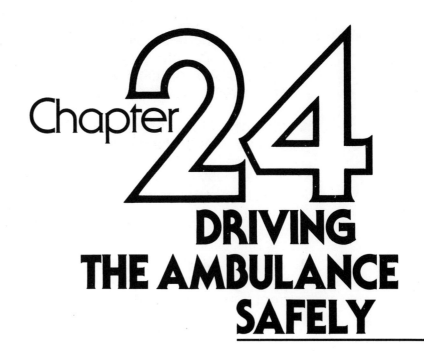

Chapter 24

DRIVING THE AMBULANCE SAFELY

Comprehensive Questions

1. Discuss the defensive driving techniques that must be employed whenever driving the ambulance.

2. Outline the procedures the ambulance driver should follow in approaching and parking at the scene of a motor vehicle accident.

3. Explain why it is necessary for the ambulance to stop at all stop signs and red lights even if it is running its lights and sirens.

Performance Skills

Safely conduct an ambulance in each of the following situations, with the proper use of lights and sirens.

1. Passing other traffic on a 2- or 4-lane highway.

2. Passing through a red light or stop sign.

3. Passing through an intersection not controlled by a traffic light.

4. Making a right or left turn at an intersection.

5. Entering and exiting a limited access highway via a ramp controlled by a stop sign.

6. Reacting to incorrect actions by drivers in response to the lights and sirens.

7. Approaching and parking at an accident scene.

Reference Data

DEFENSIVE DRIVING TECHNIQUES FOR THE AMBULANCE

1. Assume other drivers will:
   a. freeze in front of you
   b. pull out in front of you
   c. cut you off
   d. do the unexpected

2. Assume other drivers will *not*:
   a. see or hear you
   b. react properly to the ambulance
   c. obey the law

3. Never go more than 10 miles per hour over the speed limit.

4. Never exceed the speed limit in a restricted speed zone.

5. Only when using lights and sirens are you considered an emergency vehicle.

6. Remember that lights and sirens *request* the right of way; you should not take it until it is given.

7. A siren cannot be heard more than 150 feet away. Drivers will be confused as to which direction the siren is coming from.

8. Never pass vehicles on the right; drivers have been taught to pull to the right.

9. Never pass a stopped school bus in either direction until the bus driver has signaled that it is safe.

10. Park the ambulance at the accident scene so that it shields you and the patient from oncoming traffic.

Review Questions

Select the correct answer for each of the following questions. There is only *one* correct answer for each.

1. The ambulance driver is responsible for:
   a. the safety of the patient and crew.
   b. the safety of others on the road.
   c. the safe operation of the vehicle.
   d. all of the above.

2. When approaching a school bus which is displaying its flashing lights, the ambulance driver should:
   a. sound his siren and carefully pass.
   b. stop until the bus driver signals him to pass.
   c. make certain the bus is far enough to the right so that he can pass.
   d. treat the bus as any other motor vehicle.

3. Both emergency lights and sirens must be used whenever an ambulance:
   a. is responding to a call.
   b. is transporting a patient to the emergency department.
   c. is requesting the right of way or violating the motor vehicle laws.
   d. all of the above.

4. A traffic light turns red as the ambulance approaches on its way to a call. There are no vehicles in front of the ambulance. The ambulance driver should:
   a. stop, sound the siren, and proceed when safe.
   b. sound the siren, maintain speed, and proceed through.
   c. turn into a side street to avoid the light.
   d. turn off the lights and siren and wait for the light to change.

5. When CPR is being performed in the patient compartment, the ambulance should be driven at:
   a. the maximum speed road conditions and traffic allow.
   b. no more than 20 to 30 miles per hour.
   c. no more than 40 to 50 miles per hour.
   d. no more than 10 miles per hour above the posted speed limit.

6. What is the minimum distance at which an ambulance should follow another emergency vehicle?
   a. 50 feet.
   b. 100 feet.
   c. 200 feet.
   d. 300 feet.

7. An ambulance can cross a double yellow line:
    a. if traffic in both directions has pulled to the right and stopped.
    b. if the driver has a clear, unobstructed view of the road.
    c. when there are no curves or hills ahead.
    d. only if all of the above conditions are met.

8. Which of the following tasks should the ambulance driver perform before responding to a call?
    a. Adjust the seat position.
    b. Adjust the mirrors.
    c. Disconnect the charging cord.
    d. All of the above.

9. Which of the following tasks should the ambulance driver perform after returning from a call?
    a. Make certain the fuel levels are proper.
    b. Assist in replacing any used materials.
    c. Check that all emergency lights are operating properly.
    d. All of the above.

10. When approaching a stop sign with no vehicles in front of him, the ambulance driver should:
    a. sound the siren, maintain his speed, and proceed through.
    b. stop, sound the siren, and proceed when safe.
    c. proceed through, since he has the right of way.
    d. turn off the emergency lights and siren, and stop.

11. When proceeding down the right lane of a 4-lane road, with traffic on his left, the ambulance driver should:
    a. anticipate that vehicles will move to the right.
    b. sound the siren and proceed very slowly.
    c. watch for vehicles entering from the right.
    d. all of the above.

12. When approaching a red traffic light with a number of cars stopped, the ambulance driver may have to:
    a. sound the siren, move to the left lane, and pass carefully.
    b. sound the siren, and pass each car as it moves to the right.
    c. turn off the lights and sirens, and proceed as a non-emergency vehicle.
    d. radio his location and request police escort.

13. You arrive at the scene of a motor vehicle accident that occurred on a hill. The ambulance should be parked:
    a. parallel to the closest vehicle involved.
    b. on the uphill side of the scene.
    c. on the downhill side of the scene.
    d. so that it screens the scene from traffic coming in the opposite direction.

14. The ambulance must turn right at a traffic light to enter a shopping center. As it approaches, the light turns red and there are 2 lanes of vehicles stopped in front of it. The driver should:
    a. turn off the lights and sirens and proceed with the traffic.
    b. sound the siren, move into the oncoming lane, and turn into the shopping center.
    c. move into the left lane, sound the siren, and wait for the other vehicles to move right.
    d. move to the center, sound the siren, and proceed down the center as the other vehicles move left and right.

15. If a collision with another vehicle cannot be avoided, the ambulance driver should:
    a. swerve to avoid a head-on collision.
    b. turn to the right and attempt to get off the road.
    c. attempt to avoid hitting large trees or structures that appear to be permanently installed.
    d. all of the above.

16. If the use of the siren increases the anxiety of the patient, and is not absolutely necessary, the ambulance driver should:
    a. not use it and adjust his driving accordingly.
    b. disregard the patient since the law requires lights and siren.
    c. use "yelp" or "hi-lo" instead.
    d. use the horn instead.

17. Recent studies have shown that a vehicle moving in the same direction as an ambulance may not hear its siren until the ambulance is within:
    a. 25 to 35 feet.
    b. 50 to 75 feet
    c. 100 to 125 feet.
    d. 200 to 250 feet.

18. "Pre-planning" a response involves which of these actions?
    a. Knowing the road conditions.
    b. Determining the best route to the scene.
    c. Knowing the weather conditions.
    d. All of the above.

19. When approaching a traffic light that is green, the ambulance driver should:
    a. sound the siren, maintain his speed, and proceed.
    b. sound the siren, reduce his speed, and proceed.
    c. proceed as a non-emergency vehicle.
    d. sound the siren and accelerate until the intersection is cleared.

Answers to Review Questions

1: d. The ambulance driver is responsible for all of these.

2: b. The ambulance driver should stop, and proceed after the bus driver signals him to do so.

3: c. An emergency vehicle must display its lights and sound its siren whenever it operates outside the motor vehicle laws or requests right of way.

4: a. The ambulance should stop at the red light, sound its siren, and proceed only when it is safe.

5: b. Effective CPR cannot be performed in an ambulance that is traveling at more than 20 to 30 miles per hour.

6: d. An ambulance should follow another emergency vehicle at no less than 300 feet.

7: d. An ambulance can cross a double yellow line when all of these conditions are met.

8: d. All of these should be performed before responding to a call.

9: d. The ambulance driver should perform all of these tasks after returning from a call.

10: b. A stop sign should be treated the same way as a red light. The driver should stop, sound the siren, and proceed when safe.

11: d. The driver should anticipate all of these actions by other drivers.

12: c. In this situation, the driver may have to turn off the lights and siren and proceed as a non-emergency vehicle.

13: b. The ambulance should be parked uphill from an accident to avoid the possible flow of spilled gasoline.

14: a. The driver should turn off the lights and siren and proceed with the traffic.

15: d. All of these are proper defensive driving techniques if a collision is unavoidable.

16: a. The driver should discontinue the use of the siren and adjust his driving.

17: c. Studies have shown that sirens cannot be heard beyond 125 feet by a vehicle moving in the same direction.

18: d. All of these are essential parts of pre-planning a response.

19: b. The driver should sound the siren, reduce his speed, then proceed through the intersection.

Practical Applications

Consider what you would do, and why, in each of the following situations.

1. In order to reach the scene of an emergency call you must use a limited access highway. You move onto the entrance ramp, which is controlled by a stop sign, displaying the emergency lights and sounding the siren. There are 4 cars on the ramp in front of you.

2. You are responding to a motor vehicle accident on a high-traffic, 2-lane road. As you approach, the traffic is backed up about 2 miles from the scene.

3. In order to enter the shopping center you are responding to, you must make a right turn at an intersection controlled by a traffic light. As you approach, you see 2 lanes of traffic extending toward you at least one block from the traffic light.

4. The crew is performing CPR in the patient compartment. As you approach a busy intersection, the traffic light turns red.

5. You are transporting a patient that has been treated for a possible fracture of the radius and ulna. All his vital signs are in the normal range. The route to the emergency department involves passing a series of traffic lights and stop signs.

6. You are driving down a one-way street while responding to a call. Vehicles are parked on both sides of the street leaving only one lane available. There are a number of vehicles in front of you.

7. You are approximately 300 to 500 feet behind another emergency vehicle. As the first vehicle goes through an intersection, the traffic light turns red.

8. While responding to a call, you come upon the scene of a motor vehicle accident where there are several injured people.

9. While responding to a call, you are involved in a motor vehicle accident that does not disable your vehicle. There are no injuries.

Bibliography

American Academy of Orthopaedic Surgeons, Committee on Allied Health. **Emergency Care and Transportation of the Sick and Injured.** Second Edition, revised. Chicago. American Academy of Orthopaedic Surgeons, 1977.

Emergency Training. **Basic Skills for the EMT: 20 audiovisual units.** Westport, CT. Educational Direction, Inc. 1978.

Emergency Training. **Extended Skills for the EMT: The Pediatric Patient.** Westport, CT. Educational Direction, Inc. 1980.

Emergency Training. **Extended Skills for the EMT: Lifting and Moving the Patient.** Westport, CT. Educational Direction, Inc. 1980.

Emergency Training. **Extended Skills for the EMT: Using Anti-Shock Trousers (MAST).** Westport, CT. Educational Direction, Inc. 1980.

Grant, H. and Murray, R. **Emergency Care.** Second Edition. Bowie, Md. Robert J. Brady Co. 1978.

U.S. Department of Transportation. **Emergency Medical Technician-Ambulance: Basic Training Program; Course Guide and Course Coordination Orientation Program.** Washington, D.C. Government Printing Office, 1969.

About the Author

Bertram M. Siegel is Chairman of the Trumbull, Connecticut, Emergency Medical Services Commission and former Executive Director of Trumbull's EMS. As an Emergency Medical Services Instructor, he has conducted numerous training courses for EMS personnel. Mr. Siegel, who has had a long career in the field of science education, served for many years as Vice-President of Educational Direction, Inc. and with Emergency Training as a program developer and producer. His publications include books and audio-visual materials on science and emergency medical care. Mr. Siegel is a member of the National Association of Emergency Medical Technicians, the National Society of EMS Administrators, the Society of EMT Instructor-Coordinators, and the National Association of Trauma Specialists.